HOW YOU CAN BE HEALED TODAY

OF

CANCER, AIDS or OTHER AFFLICTIONS

BY

THE GIFT OF HEALING

With Instructions On How You Can Be Healed
And Stay Healed

BY

ROBERT L. BUFKIN

HOW YOU CAN BE HEALED TODAY

OF CANCER, AIDS OR OTHER AFFLICTIONS

by

THE GIFT OF HEALING

With Instructions On How You Can Be Healed and STAY Healed

Published by
'fishers of men' Church
WORLD MISSIONARY OUTREACH

Robert L. Bufkin Ministries
PO Box 17382
Jonesboro AR 72403

http://www.rlbm.org
anelijah@fastmail.fm

First Printing   July 1955
Twenty-second revision and printing   March 2008
23rd Revision and Printing September 2009
24th Revision December 2009

CONTENTS

I AM ONLY A STEWARD OVER ANOTHER MAN'S VALUABLE TREASURE.

All this really means is that I have been entrusted by the Lord Jesus with a valuable treasure, The Gift of Healing, and must one day give account to the Master. My consuming passion is to administer this Gift around the world to all people who will believe. I can truly say with awe and reverence as I minister to the sick and suffering, the Lord is stretching forth his hand to heal, Acts 4:29-30 just like he did in Bible days. See also Mark 16:20.

MY PERSONAL DISCLAIMER

I am not a healer. I speak the words the Lord Jesus gave me to say, but Jesus alone does the healing. John 14:12, Jesus said that his followers would do the same works that he did, because he is going to the Father and send another comforter - the Holy Ghost. Then in Acts I :8, Jesus said, "You shall receive power after that the Holy Ghost is come upon you and you shall be witnesses unto me. Any healing that takes place is the work of the Spirit of Christ, the Lord Jesus alone.

MY MANDATE

In 1 Peter 4:10 (TEV) is my mandate, "Each one, as a good manager of God's different gifts, must use for the good of others the special gift he has received from God"

Mark 16:20. The followers went everywhere in the world and told the Good News to people, and the Lord helped them. The Lord proved that the Good News they told was true by giving them power to work miracles. (NCV)

I can say as Jesus taught me to say, If I do not the works of my Father, believe me not. But if people are really healed of cancer and aids and other demonic oppression instantly by my command, then believe me for the very works sake. The Father who dwells in me, he does the works. I Cor. 3:16; 6:19-20; John 10:37-38; 14:10-12.

"The words that I speak unto you I speak not of myself: my Father gave me these words to say and I speak even as he has commanded and he alone does the works of healing and forgiving sins."

But be assured that Jesus Christ never healed anyone apart from their faith or believing in him. The Gift of Jesus for healing does not work by magic or witch craft methods but by hearing the Word, then believing that Word and acting on that Word.

So you must listen to the two truths about the Cross and the Whipping Post and believe it with all your heart. The simplicity of the Gospel has been so perverted and corrupted and overshadowed by religion and tradition of denominations and rituals that many people know little about the real genuine basic truths about the Cross of Jesus Christ, what he really accomplished there and about the whipping he took just before the Cross.

The Gift of Healing will only work if you first hear the genuine simple truth about the Cross and the Whipping Post. Then your faith will be released from fear and hopelessness and guilt and rise up to strike cancer or sickness out of your life and keep it out.

Jesus never healed anyone apart from faith. The following sections will build your faith in the healing power of Jesus Christ. You will see Jesus Christ as deity and as the image of God and as the resurrected Christ. You will see him as a present help today. For when he rose from the dead and ascended into heaven, he sent the Holy Ghost, who is called the Spirit of Christ seven times in the New Testament.

The Spirit of Christ is present with you right where you are right now as you read these words. Open your heart and believe the truths presented here from the Bible and your faith will increase to the point that you can and will be healed. This is the Gift of Healing, not anointing with oil, not the prayer of faith, not two agreeing together, but the Gift of Healing at work. No disease or demon can stand against the operation of the Gift of Healing. That is why so many thousands world wide have been healed instantly of nearly every disease and affliction known to man. You're next. Get ready.

HOW THE GIFT OF HEALING CAME INTO MY LIFE

The doctor said, "Your wife is terminal with cancer, and she will die about October 20, 1985". That was in March 1985. The world came crashing down around me. I couldn't accept what the doctor said. But my wife, Annette, died on October 17, 1985.

I LEARNED TO HATE CANCER

Then my older daughter, Patricia, got cancer and died 17 months later. I saw these two beautiful Spirit filled people turned into withered shells. I saw cancer victims constantly at the hospital in all stages of the disease. I already feared cancer, but I now learned to hate cancer. I saw cancer as a living thing, a diabolical mind holding the entire human race hostage to fear. I saw cancer like a pack of savage wolves chasing men, women and children, attacking babies and mothers; all races and all classes of people. I wept every day for four and a half months.

THE GIFTS OF HEALING

Then I read, 1 Corinthians 12:9,10 where Jesus set Gifts of Healing in the Spirit filled church. My prayer became, "Lord I want the Gift of Healing that heals cancer and AIDS instantly", and he gave it to me after much fasting and prayer.

WEEKS OF FASTING AND PRAYER

First there was a 21 day fast. Then many shorter fasts. Finally on the last day of August 1989, I began a consecration fast unto the Lord and went to an Ozark Mountain cabin. I stayed with the consecration until October 13, 1989. For forty-three days I sought the Lord for the Gift of Healing that heals all forms of cancer and AIDS. During the sixth week of that fast the presence of the Lord filled the cabin like a golden glow. I felt his presence in a very special way as I lay flat of my back on a little bunk. Then Jesus appeared to me. I saw him from the waist up. I saw his face and I heard his voice during those two days and two nights.

First the Lord just looked at me for a long while. Then I realized that something wonderful had happened.
He had taken away the fear of cancer and AIDS. He spoke very slowly and told me not to pray for the sick. Then he said, "I never prayed for the sick." He showed me that the Gift of Healing doesn't operate by praying for people. He told me to call the demon by name, bind it in Jesus' Name then command it to come out and it will go instantly.

The Gift works by speaking - not praying. I had not asked for prayer power but for the Gift of Healing and the Gift does not work by prayer. Multitudes have been healed by asking in prayer. It happens all the time. See Matthew 18:19; 21:22 and James 5: 14-15. I had asked for the Gift of healing and the gift works by Words of instruction to focus faith on the Lord Jesus Christ.

The Lord showed me that the word 'GIFT' used in 1 Corinthians in the Authorized King James version, which is the Greek word 'charisma' means: A bright light, indicating the presence of deity. This is the presence of the Holy Ghost, God in us. The light that shown from the face of Jesus on the Mount of Transfiguration indicated that all the fullness of deity dwelt in him. That Shekinah Glory was: a bright light indicating the presence of deity.

In 2 Corinthians 4:4-6, "The light of the Glory of God is in the face of Jesus Christ". The nine gifts of the Spirit, listed in 1 Corinthians 12:7-11, indicate the presence of Jesus working through his Body, the Church, to continue his wonderful saving and healing ministry in the earth.

Then the Lord Jesus told me these exact words: "Cancer is not a germ disease, cancer is a devil." Then the Lord Jesus told me to tell people two things ... one thing about the Cross and one thing about the whipping he took. If they will believe this and make a simple confession of faith, then the cancer devil will come out when I speak the words he gave me and they will be healed. All I do is call the spirit by name, bind it using the name Jesus Christ and command it to come out and it goes. It really works. Read and believe and you too can be healed and delivered from demon oppression, aids, cancer or any affliction. See Acts 10:38.

IS IT NECESSARY TO HAVE FAITH?

Without faith it is impossible to please God. "All who come to God must believe (have faith)" Heb. 11:6.

Jesus said, "Go thy way, as thou hast believed so be it done unto thee:" Matt. 8:13. Jesus never healed by caprice or whim. He always required faith on the part of the sick. It doesn't take super faith, but it does take faith.
The only time Jesus did not heal was, because of their unbelief, Mark6:5-6. Jesus said, "If you can believe, all things are possible to them that believe," Mark 9:23. But without faith it is impossible.

NEVER CALL IT "MY CANCER" AGAIN

You must stop going over your symptoms in your speech and thoughts. Never again tell anyone where you hurt or anything about your physical condition and never describe your treatment to anyone. Abraham was strong in faith for one reason, he considered not his own body, but instead he considered only what the Word of God said about his body, Romans 4:19.

Notice this promise, "Whosoever offers praise, glorifieth me: and to him that ordereth his conversation aright will I show the salvation of God", (Psalms 50:23). You must take charge of your speech and stop talking doubt and symptoms and what the doctor said. You must talk Bible talk. Say what God says about you, "BY HIS STRIPES I AM HEALED. HE HEALETH ALL MY DISEASES. JESUS TOOK ALL MY SICKNESS." If you confess his Word he will show you his salvation, and not before. Begin ordering your speech to reflect what the WORD says and not what your body or doctor or others say.

PUT JESUS TO WORK FOR YOU AND STOP LICENSING SATAN AND DOUBT

Jesus said, "If you will confess me before men, I will confess you before the throne of Heaven". Matt. 10:31-32. Put Jesus to work confessing your name in Heaven. Only you can do that. Jesus, is our high priest, he is waiting at the blood stained altar in heaven to hear your confession. If you confess the right thing - HIS WORDS AND HIS PRAISE - He will confess your name before that blood stained altar. Put Jesus to work for you now. Remember, there are two forces in the world each trying to get your attention, Jesus and satan. Your confession licenses one of them. License Jesus today and every day. Never again license pain and disease and satan and doubt and defeat. Confess God's words about healing and you will be on firm safe ground to keep your healing.

A WORD ABOUT SYMPTOMS

Once healed of cancer, most people find the first three days after their healing to be the most difficult. The cancer which has been eating on their body is now dead. So their body begins to eat away at the dead tumor cells. This will cause some feeling of nausea which will last for about 3 days more or less. But that is not the cancer; it is a sign of your healing. Most people notice a difference in the pain immediately when I take my hands off their head, saying "come out". The pain either leaves completely the first day or it diminishes until it is gone after a short time. And they sleep much better the very first night after their healing. Confess loudly MY DAILY CONFESSIONS on pg. 85, twice daily and faith and joy will surge through your spirit.

The organs of your body absorbed the deadly chemicals you received from the cancer treatment. Now that the cancer is dead, your bodily organs begin to throw the deadly chemicals back into your system a little at a time so your body can dispose of the material through the regular channels of elimination. This may give you **'flashbacks'** of dizziness or nausea or pain. Don't be fearful of this discomfort. It is a sign of healing.

WHEN THE SUN GOES DOWN - - FEVERS GO UP!

In the darkness and stillness of night the mind begins to wander. If you should have any symptom of fear or pain at night or anytime, open this book and affirm aloud the words of healing on pgs. 18-22, again and again. Speak to your mountain - the fear or symptom- and command it to leave in Jesus Name and it will go. Be sure to confess your Daily Confession Sheet twice daily for 21 days, (Pg 39). It will transform your life if you keep it up and force yourself to say it. Your faith will grow very strong.

THE SOCIAL FACTORS OF FAITH AND DOUBT

Your faith or doubt is a direct reflection of the faith or doubt of your parents and your community of reference. If your parents and church did not believe in miracles and taught against miracles for today, then you will believe the same thing. If you get healed by this Gift of Healing and then go back into a non-believing church and support a preacher who preaches against miracles such as you have received, you dishonor the Lord Jesus who has healed you and you open the way for demons of cancer or illness to come back in your body. Call me, I can find you a believing church to attend. John 5:1-14.

HINDRANCES TO YOUR FAITH AND HOW TO KEEP YOUR HEALING

Don't let your community of unbelief talk you out of your miracle. You must remove all hindrances to your faith. I'll help you remove all hindrances as we go to prayer and healing later in the book.

Here is a short list of things that will hinder your faith and even kill your faith. **Remove them from your life** and you will grow in the Lord and your faith will remain strong.

Holding sin in your heart, Ps. 66:18; Prov. 28:13;
Lukewarmness, Rev. 3:15,16;

An unforgiving attitude toward your enemies and those that hurt you, Matt. 6:15; 5:23,24;
Looking at your symptoms instead of the word, Rom. 4: 18-21,
Not confessing your healing to everyone, Matt. 10:32,33, Heb.10:35;
If your heart condemns you, 1 John 3:32;   (by not repenting of all sin)
Not giving honor to your spouse, 1 Peter 3:7.

Check off each hindrance to faith on the list as you win the victory over it. Repent of all your sins daily and ask the Lord Jesus to forgive you. Forgive your enemies daily. Open your heart and let them go. It takes practice to really forgive your enemies.

FAMILY PARTICIPATION IS NECESSARY

When Jesus raised Lazarus from the dead, he gave a command to the loved ones of Lazarus, "Loose him and let him go". Wound tightly in the wrappings of the grave clothes, Lazarus couldn't eat, drink or do anything associated with life. Let me ask you, how long would Lazarus have lived if someone had not helped him after his miracle by unwinding the grave clothes so he could be free? Jesus' great miracle would have failed utterly in a few hours without family participation.

Yes, Lazarus would have died again if someone had not helped him immediately after his resurrection. It lies in your power, loved one, to help nourish and love the former cancer victim back to health and create in them a strong will to live and a desire to re-enter life. It took family participation to complete the miracle of Lazarus' resurrection. Help complete your loved ones miracle by giving love, a nourishing diet and exercise and faith.

Get my book on, THE NATURE OF FAITH and THE BLIND SPOT OF MEDICAL DOCTORS. It will build your faith even more. Many have said it is the most helpful book in print on having faith for miracles.

CANCER OFTEN GETS IN THROUGH THE WOUND OF A BROKEN HEART

Cancer is a social relationship disease. It is now known that the human brain exercises full control over the body's immune system. Therefore, Medical Scientists claim that if you get cancer, you had to give it permission to work in your body, but at the subconscious level. Scientists believe that great emotional stress can cause the immune system to be suppressed and trigger cancer cells to begin growing. So, whatever causes you great stress can sponsor cancer in your body. Many cancer victims have written an emotional script which reads like a suicide note: "I am causing my loved ones pain", so I will die and get out of their way so they can be happy.

Cancer is your way of agreeing with your worst opinion about yourself. Medical Science says that you can't get cancer without your permission. So withdraw permission for cancer to work in your body. Say it out loud.

I am fighting for your life. Won't you join me with all your heart? If you do, nothing will keep you from being healed and staying healed. The God that answers by fire, let him be your God from this day.

Another study found that many cancer victims felt they were unwanted as children. So their suicide script includes the message that they are finally giving into their parent's wishes. Cancer is your way of agreeing with their worst opinion about yourself. Cancer has been called the disease of 'nice' people, who often put the interest of others ahead of their own. Most unhappy people can't divorce or commit suicide for one reason or another so the victim sees cancer as the only honorable way out, albeit the most painful. Doctors call this, 'benign' suicide. Sadly, it is common among cancer patients. They refuse to fight back. They actually have a wish to die. So when I come against cancer, I am coming against the entire negative past of the victim and their negative 'self-destruct' mind-set they developed over years of unhappiness.

Now, consider this: a broken heart predisposed you to cancer. So when your cancer is healed, you must then deal with the negative, self-destructive emotions still lurking in your memory system from the broken heart; else your predisposition to cancer will arise and strike yet again. You must find a new way of responding to the stress that opened the door to cancer. I will show you how to do that

How do you heal a broken heart? Get in a Spirit filled church and receive the Baptism of the Holy Ghost as in Acts 2:4; 10:46-47; and 19:1-7. Worship the Lord Jesus Christ and sing praises to him with all your heart. Learn to forgive all your enemies and everyone who has ever hurt you. Confess the Daily Confession Sheet in the back of this book. Say it loudly twice a day for 21 days and it will transform your life. Call or write me. I will help you find a Spirit filled church.

If you don't forgive those who have hurt you, then the wounds they caused will most likely become like a shrine in your memory with a life all it's own. That shrine will then speak hate and vengeance and self pity to you day and night and will color all your words, thoughts and actions: thereby keeping the old wound open and fresh and bleeding. Enter cancer!

Forgiving your enemy, who wounded you, in the Name of the Lord Jesus, is the only way to allow healing to begin; thus closing up those wounds and denying cancer an opening into your life. You must forgive yourself and all your enemies. You may feel it necessary to even forgive God, if you blame Him for letting your enemy wound you or allowing some other tragedy to happen in your life.

When the doctor looks at you and says, "You have cancer", fear stabs your heart. Cancer is a death sentence. Next you begin seeing a world without yourself. Then the death sentence grows into the death wish, which finally matures into the will to die. If you don't want to live, no help from God or man will bring you healing. Looking at the Cross and believing that Jesus Christ loved you enough to take all you sins into his own body on the tree and then suffer the death blow those sins deserved; thereby paying the full price for your sins; will help you see and feel his love for you. Looking at the Cross will instill in you the truth of your real value and worth as a human being. Jesus Christ really is alive and he really does love you more than you ever have been loved in your life. Accept his love. Open your heart to him. Invite him to come in and he will make you know you are loved. He will heal the wounds and give you a sense of purpose in life and the will to live. He will never force you to live. Only the Blood of Jesus Christ can cleanse from sin and guilt and from hatred. Call on the Name of Jesus right now and ask him to forgive you and cleanse you from sin and guilt and old wounds and baptize you with the Holy Ghost. He will answer your prayer. Whosoever shall call upon the Name of the Lord shall be saved. Call today.

HOW TO HAVE FAITH FOR HEALING OR ANY MIRACLE

Healing for the physical body has always been an integral part of the relationship between Jehovah God and mankind. There has never been a period of time in history called, 'the age of miracles'. A miracle is defined as any act of God that changes the natural order of things. All the way from Genesis to Malachi, forty-two different names and titles were applied to Jehovah God. One of the most prominent names God gave himself was Jehovah-Rapha or the Lord our Healer.

Keep this in mind at all times: If you want to be healed in your body by the Lord Jesus, you must forsake all other gods and goddesses and religions and preachers and holy men or woman or objects or images or idols and religious beliefs and doctrines and cling to the Lord Jesus and him only and to what he taught as recorded by the only eye witnesses who lived with him day and night for over three years. The eye witnesses knew the full truth. Listen to them and live as they speak in the Book of Acts where they began their ministry to the world.

Jesus commissioned those eye witnesses, <u>and no one else</u>, to teach the entire world exactly what he had taught them. All that Jesus commanded for us to believe is recorded by those eye witnesses in the Bible, which is only sixty-six books, from Genesis to Malachi and from Matthew to the book of Revelation. Their teaching began in the Book of Acts.

Jehovah God has healed sicknesses from the beginning of creation. We read from the Old Testament, examples of God's healing power at work in the lives of sick and afflicted human beings.

THE KING OF GERAR HEALED BY FAITH

In Gen 20:7, "Now therefore restore the man his wife; for he is a prophet, and he shall pray for thee, and thou shalt live: and if thou restore her not, know thou that thou shalt surely die, thou, and all that are thine."

Abimelech, the King of Gerar, had taken Abraham's wife, Sarah, into his harem intending to marry her. But the Lord struck all of Abimelech's household with a plague because of that sinful act. The Lord told Abimelech to restore Abraham's wife to him or else he would die.

Notice that the Lord told the King if he would restore Sarah to her husband then Abraham would pray for him and the Lord promised to heal the King and all his household. "So Abraham prayed unto God: and God healed Abimelech, and his wife, and his maidservants; and they bare children." (Gen 20:17 KJV)

Healing of the sick and afflicted in answer to the prayer of a righteous man brought healing for a King and his entire household. Nothing has changed about God's healing power for sick and suffering mankind.

NAAMAN THE SYRIAN GENERAL HEALED BY FAITH

Next we hear Jehovah claiming to be a healer. No man, no doctor, and no preacher is a healer who can heal instantly by supernatural means. Only the living God can heal instantly by supernatural means.

"See now that I, even I, am he, and there is no god with me: I kill, and I make alive; I wound, and I heal: neither is there any that can deliver out of my hand." (Deut. 32:39 KJV)

When Naaman the Syrian was struck with leprosy, a little Hebrew slave girl who worked in his kitchen told him that a prophet in Israel could recover him of his leprosy. The fact that a child knew that her God, Jehovah, worked miracles of physical healing through a prophet shows that healing for the body was common knowledge and practice in Israel thousands of years ago.

Naaman went to Israel and found that prophet and after dipping seven times in the river Jordan was completely healed of his leprosy. Jehovah is a Healer; always has been and always will be.

HEZEKIAH HEALED BY FAITH

Here is another case of healing in answer to prayer. Hezekiah the King was sick unto death. He was praying for healing from the Lord. The prophet told the King, to set his house in order for he would die of his disease. But then Hezekiah prayed earnestly and the Lord heard his plea for healing and told the prophet, "Turn again, and tell Hezekiah the captain of my people, Thus saith the LORD, the God of David thy father, I have heard thy prayer, I have seen thy tears: behold, I will heal thee: on the third day thou shalt go up unto the house of the LORD." (2 Ki 20:5 KJV)

Another promise of healing by the power of God supernaturally, "If my people, which are called by my name, shall humble themselves, and pray, and seek my face, and turn from their wicked ways; then will I hear from heaven, and will forgive their sin, and will heal their land." (2 Chr 7:14 KJV)

Here is a short list of scriptures which speak of God the Healer, healing sick bodies.

- "And ye shall serve the LORD your God, and he shall bless thy bread, and thy water; and I will take sickness away from the midst of thee." (Exo 23:25 KJV)

- "And the LORD will take away from thee all sickness, and will put none of the evil diseases of Egypt, which thou knowest, upon thee; but will lay them upon all them that hate thee." Deu 7:15 (KJV)

- "For I will restore health unto thee, and I will heal thee of thy wounds, saith the LORD; because they called thee an Outcast, saying, This is Zion, whom no man seeketh after." (Jer 30:17 KJV)

- "O LORD my God, I cried unto thee, and thou hast healed me." (Psa 30:2 KJV)

- "He sent his word, and healed them, and delivered them from their destructions." (Psa 107:20 KJV)

- "But he was wounded for our (DISEASES), he was bruised for our (SICKNESSES): the chastisement of our peace was upon him; and with his stripes we are healed." (Isa 53:5 KJV) (The proper translation is, diseases and sicknesses)

- Note that Peter quotes this same verse in 1 Peter 2:24b, and with his stripes ye were healed.

GOD'S NAME… (hence his NATURE)…IS HEALER!

And here is the most amazing commandment of the Lord. He gives mankind his name, Jehovah-Rapha. So healing for the physical bodies of sick and afflicted human beings is Almighty God's name, and therefore a permanent part of his NATURE. And God never changes and in fact cannot change. He never changes his Name; or his nature. Healer is what God is and therefore is what God does.

"If thou wilt diligently hearken to the voice of the LORD thy God, and wilt do that which is right in his sight, and wilt give ear to his commandments, and keep all his statutes, I will put none of these diseases upon thee, which I have brought upon the Egyptians: for I am the LORD that healeth thee." (Exo 15:26 KJV)

"Bless the LORD, O my soul, and forget not all his benefits: Who forgiveth all thine iniquities; who healeth all thy diseases", (Psa 103:2,3 KJV) But remember the Lord said, do not forget all his benefits. He not only forgives all sin but he heals all our sicknesses. If you forget his benefits it's the same as if there were no benefits.

And in the New Testament, Jesus spent a great deal of time healing large masses of people all over Palestine. We read the words, "and great multitudes followed him and he healed them all." Yes, Jesus was the Word in person. In Christ Jesus, Jehovah had sent his Word and healed the people.

JESUS CREATED HIS CHURCH BY THE POWER OF THE HOLY GHOST BAPTISM

Also we notice that Jesus Christ created the Church and called it "my church" in Matthew 16:18. It was the power of the Baptism of the Holy Ghost and fire that was given on the Day of Pentecost that created the Body of Christ.

At the very beginning of his ministry, John the Baptist had promised the Jesus would baptize people with the Holy Ghost. Then at the close of Jesus' ministry he promised the disciples that, "For John truly baptized with water; but ye shall be baptized with the Holy Ghost not many days hence." (Acts 1:5 KJV). So seven days later on the Day of Pentecost, the Holy Ghost fell on the 120 and they were Baptized or Filled with the Holy Ghost and they all spoke in other languages as the Spirit gave them the utterance. That baptism birthed the Body of Christ on earth and gave gifts to them by that power of the Holy Ghost which is power over all the power of demons and sickness.

JESUS HANDED OUT THE POWER TO HEAL TO MEN

Now when Jesus ascended on high and sat down at the right hand of God, he poured out the Holy Ghost baptism and thereby distributed a Baptismal measure of the fullness of deity which dwelt in him. Jesus gave gifts unto men beginning at that time. The scripture says that Jesus ascended above all things that he might fill all things. So it was the Spirit of Jesus that filled the 120 and he gave gifts to them. He still gives gifts to every man he baptizes with the Holy Ghost. 1 Cor.12:7,11.

"Wherefore he saith, when he ascended up on high, he led captivity captive, and gave gifts unto men."

"He that descended is the same also that ascended up far above all heavens, that he might fill all things."

"And he gave some, apostles; and some, prophets; and some, evangelists; and some, pastors and teachers;"

"For the perfecting of the saints, for the work of the ministry, for the edifying of the body of Christ:"

"Till we all come in the unity of the faith, and of the knowledge of the Son of God, unto a perfect man, unto the measure of the stature of the fullness of Christ: {So those gifts are still here today} That we henceforth be no more children, tossed to and fro, and carried about with every wind of doctrine, by the sleight of men, and cunning craftiness, whereby they lie in wait to deceive." (Eph 4:8-14 KJV)

The gifts mentioned here are offices of authority denoting different ministries given to men and the purpose of founding and directing churches and teaching doctrine. As long as there is a Church, those offices are still present and are ordained of the Lord Jesus for the good of his Church until he comes back to earth again.

THESE GIFTS ARE FOR EVERY MEMBER OF THE BODY OF CHRIST

But the gifts listed in 1 Cor. 12:7-11 are for every member of the Body of Christ and include a gift of Healing and a gift of Miracles. "But the manifestation of the Spirit is given to every man to profit withal. For to one is given by the Spirit the word of wisdom; to another the word of knowledge by the same Spirit; To another faith by the same Spirit; to another the gifts of healing by the same Spirit; To another the working of miracles; to another prophecy; to another discerning of spirits; to another divers kinds of tongues; to another the interpretation of tongues: But all these worketh that one and the selfsame Spirit, dividing to every man severally as he will." (1 Cor 12:7-11 KJV)

The word 'gifts' is 'charisma' in the Greek and means, 'a bright light, indicating the presence of deity.' The nine operations or manifestations of the Spirit of Christ listed in 1 Cor. 12: 8-10, are in truth the Lord Jesus himself living and acting through his Body the Church to continue his powerful ministry in the earth. Three gifts to know, three to act, and three to speak - like the Lord Jesus.

The gift of Healing is for the supernatural healing of human sicknesses. The gift of Miracles is for power over demon spirits to cast them out. Many of the afflictions of mankind are caused by the presence of demon spirits of infirmity. The gift of Faith is in operation for power over nature and inanimate objects or afflictions.

As long as there is a Body of Christ on the earth, there will be these nine manifestations of the Spirit of Christ working in and through the lives of that Body. Jesus set these gifts and callings and ministries in "his church" and they cannot pass away, just as the Church cannot pass away. Jesus said, "My words shall never pass away".

It is vital to remember that the mighty Baptism of the Holy Ghost and the powerful gifts of the Spirit were all poured out by the resurrected Jesus to create the Body of Christ on earth. (Acts 2:33) It took power to create new creatures. "But as many as received him, to them gave he <u>power to become the sons of God</u>, even to them that believe on his name: Which were born, not of blood, nor of the will of the flesh, nor of the will of man, but of God." (John 1:12,13 KJV). Jesus said, "You shall receive POWER after the Holy Ghost is come upon you…".Acts 1:8. And again 2 Cor. 5:17 says, If any man be IN CHRIST he is a New Creation….

And every member of that Body in the Book of Acts was a human being just like you and me. But the gifts of position (offices) and power (9 gifts) which the Lord Jesus gave were to over-ride their humanness by recreating them in the image of Jesus himself by the born again experience and to manifest himself to the world through their lives and ministries, for the purpose of continuing his beautiful ministry in the earth. Selah!

Jesus gave them abilities to know supernaturally, to speak supernaturally and to act supernaturally by the power that works within them. (Eph. 3:20),"He is able to do exceedingly above all that we ask or thing, <u>according to the power that works in us</u>." Those gifts and abilities are in truth the Spirit of the Lord Jesus himself living in "his Church", the fullness of him that filleth all in all. "And hath put all things under his feet, and gave him to be the head over all things <u>to the church</u>, Which is his body, <u>the fullness of him that filleth all in all</u>." (Eph 1:22,23 KJV)

JESUS CHRIST IS NOW THE POWER CENTER OF THE UNIVERSE

Jesus is the power center of the universe. "All power both in heaven and earth is given unto me." Matthew 28:18) In him dwells all the fullness of the God nature bodily. (Col. 2:9) I saw ALL in ALL when I saw Jesus Christ.

JESUS DELEGATED THAT POWER TO MERE MEN

But it was a vesting from without - not a power within. In the beginning of the Lord's earthly ministry he called a group of twelve men and sent them out to preach the Gospel of the Kingdom of God. And he delegated some of that power to them and gave them power to cast out devils, heal the sick and raise the dead. "Behold, I give unto you power to tread on serpents and scorpions, and over all the power of the enemy: and nothing shall by any means hurt you." (Luke 10:19 KJV) The twelve went out and preached the Gospel and cast out devils by using the Name of the Lord Jesus. Mark told it this way: "And he ordained twelve, that they should be with him, and that he might send them forth to preach, And to have power to heal sicknesses, and to cast out devils:" (Mark 3:14,15 KJV)

Then Jesus called and appointed seventy more men and sent them out two by two and gave them power over the devil and to cure diseases. "Behold, I give unto you power to tread on serpents and scorpions, and over all the power of the enemy: and nothing shall by any means hurt you." (Luke 10:19 KJV)

THE RESURRECTED JESUS GIVES OUT GIFTS TO HEAL AND WORK MIRACLES TO MEN THROUGH THEIR NEW NATURE RECEIVED BY THE BAPTISM OF THE HOLY GHOST AS IN ACTS 2:4.

But after Jesus rose from the dead, thus certifying the nature and identity and power of his shed Blood, he ascended into the heavens and sat down at the right hand of God. He had all power in heaven and earth and a Name above every name in heaven (even Jehovah) and earth, in this world and in to the world to come. From that exalted position Jesus poured out the Baptism of the Holy Ghost. On the Day of Pentecost, Peter explained, "Jesus, (whom you crucified) has poured forth this which you now see and hear." Acts 2:33. The first two groups of ministers, the 12 and the 70, which Jesus sent out had a commission or a vesting of power to carry out their ministry among men. That power was external.

But now, the resurrected Christ acting from his position as the power center of the universe actually 'possessed' the physical bodies of the 120 waiting souls on the Day of Pentecost and performed a new birth within making them the children of God by faith in Jesus

Christ, i.e. the Body of Christ on earth. How did he do this? By his Spirit. The first man Adam was made a living soul. How? By the Spirit of Jehovah which he breathed into the body of Adam. The Spirit produces sonship. But the last Adam (Jesus Christ) was made life giving Spirit. 1 Cor. 15:45.

You see that healing power for the physical body is a very wonderful and permanent part of God's dealing with human beings in all ages. In the Old Testament there were many promises of healing for sickness given by the Lord himself. And, as we have seen, there were many examples of God healing sick bodies by supernatural means.

JESUS PAID FOR OUR SINS BY HIS SHED BLOOD; THEN HEALS US OF SICKNESS BY HIS STRIPES

Then in the New Testament, healing for the physical body became a covenant right for all the Body of Christ by the stripes that fell upon the Lord Jesus. Jesus bought and paid for physical healing for believers. Jesus called his healing power, "the children's bread". To say that the blood shed at Calvary for our sin is more important than the beating he suffered for our physical healing, begs the issue. Of course the Blood of Jesus shed for our sins at the Cross is all important. But we must never forget all his benefits which include healing for the body as well as forgiveness of sins.

JESUS IS TOUCHED WITH THE FEELING OF OUR INFIRMITIES - HE FEELS WHAT WE FEEL.

Jesus said, "somebody hath touched me: for I perceive that virtue is gone out of me." (Luke 8:46 KJV) The word 'virtue' is the same word as 'power' in Acts 1:8. Power is gone out of me is what Jesus was saying.

Why? Because in this case only one person in that multitude reached out in faith and touched his garment. Only faith in the Lord Jesus can draw upon his healing virtue. But where a person with faith touches him, it is as though his healing virtue is set on automatic, that virtue immediately goes out of Jesus into the body of the sick and heals all sickness. No sickness or affliction can resist the virtue of Jesus, if the seeker has faith.

In the Old Testament, unclean had the power. If an unclean person touched a clean person, the uncleanness went immediately into the clean person making them also unclean immediately. But Jesus reversed the curse. Clean had come to walk among mankind. When unclean touched Jesus, clean went out of him and cleaned up the unclean. Glory!

Our needs drew our God (in Christ) to us to save and heal us. He is touched with the feeling of our infirmities so our physical hurts, hurt the Lord Jesus. He feels our pains. Matt. 8:17, See also Isaiah 63:9 says, "In all their affliction, He (Jehovah) was afflicted." He is touched with the feeling of what hurts us. Isn't that a wonderful Jesus?

HERE IS HOW TO USE YOUR FAITH RIGHT NOW FOR YOUR HEALING

Faith means you believe something has happened even before you see it happen. Faith means you believe something you cannot prove. We walk by faith and not by sight. So faith and sight are at opposite polls. Therefore if you have to see something before you believe it, then you are not using faith at all. You are walking by sight and not faith. For example, when Mary and Martha came out to see Jesus four days after the funeral of their brother Lazarus, they said they believed Lazarus would rise from the dead at the last day. But listen to what Jesus said. "I am the resurrection." - meaning that Jesus was deity with all power over death and the grave. But then when the sisters doubted, Jesus said, "Did not I tell you that if you would believe, you should see the glory of God."

If you believe, you shall see. If you believe you shall see. But the natural carnal mind says, only if I see, will I believe for "seeing is believing." But Jesus says, "Believing is seeing". So sight and faith are opposites of each other. Sight is not in the nature of faith. Faith does not use eyes or the human senses. Faith accepts only what the WORD of GOD says and not what the eyes and physical senses say.

One day Jehovah told Joshua to look across the River Jordan and see the city of Jericho with its hundred foot high walls. Then he said, "Joshua, I have given you the city." But there it was still standing with hundred foot high walls and fortified, and Joshua and the nation of Israel still on the other side of Jordan. But Joshua believed the Word of the Lord and rejoiced over the victory, even before the battle took place. That's faith. Joshua confessed, the victory is ours even before they went into battle. That's faith. The evidence of things not seen. Not seen. Not seen. That's the nature of faith. Looking at the invisible. They endured as, "seeing him who is invisible". Glory! That's how you will win also.

So faith didn't depend on sight. In fact sight and faith just don't mix. If you have to see something in order to believe it, then you are canceling Jesus and faith altogether. You must believe it because the Word of God said it, even before the promise appears fulfilled before you or within you. Believe and you shall see the glory of God is what Jesus teaches. Jesus said, when you pray, believe you receive it and you shall have it. Believing is receiving, before seeing comes into view. Mark 11:24 (ASV) Therefore I say unto you, All things whatsoever ye pray and ask for, believe that ye receive them, and ye shall have them. Shall have is future tense. Faith believes you have something before you see it in reality.

That is why the Bible says that faith comes by hearing the Word of God. The Word of God gives the promises and tells how the Lord carries out those promises in every case without one failure. That builds faith in a person to believe God's Words of promise and to believe the promises will work for him also.

"(T)here hath not failed one word of all his good promise, which he promised by the hand of Moses his servant." (1 Ki 8:56 K
"Then said the LORD unto me, ... I will hasten (stand behind) my word to perform it." (Jer 1:12 KJV)

God is not a man that he should lie, hath he said and shall he not do it; or hath he spoken and shall he not make it good. Numbers 23:19.

So shall my word be that goes forth out of my mouth; it shall not return unto me void but it shall accomplish the thing I sent it to do. Isaiah 55:11.

YOU HAVE FAITH – HERE'S HOW YOU CAN USE IT AND BE HEALED

All faith begins with knowledge. You hear the statements put forth by the Lord God and by his prophets and apostles. Next comes believing that knowledge. Last comes the action required by that knowledge you have just believed. But all three work together to project the image we call faith. You read the many scriptures where the Lord God gives his very name as Healer along with all his promises to heal the sick. Then you read of all the innumerable miracles of healing the Lord performed as recorded in scripture. Next you read and hear about all the many miracles of healing that have taken place in your world of today.

Then you make a decision that changes your life forever. You either decide to believe those facts or to disbelieve those facts. There is no middle ground. If you believe those facts, then you act accordingly.

THE POINT, THE PERIOD AND THE ACTION LAW

We find here a law. The law of the point, the period and the action. A point with regard to time and place. A period with regard to confession. And an action with regard to perfection.

1. <u>Faith always sets a time and place to act</u>. When I touch the border of his garment I shall be whole. When I dip seven times in the Jordan River I shall be healed. When hands are laid on me I shall be healed. When the cloth that once touched the body of the apostle Paul, is laid on my body, demons and disease will come out. Faith always sets a time and place to act. Before that time, you are sick. At that point, your sickness leaves. After that point, you are no longer sick.

2. <u>Faith always puts a period to hopes confession</u>. Faith stops saying I hope so; or maybe so; and starts saying I know I have been

healed. Faith confesses that Bible verse that says, by his stripes I am healed, regardless of circumstances. Regardless of all 'signs' to the contrary, faith confesses what the Word of God says instead of what their body says. Your circumstances then conform to your confession. Have the faith of God. God spoke and it came into being. Be imitators of God as dear children. Speak his word about your case and it will come into being. Romans 4:17, He calls those things that be not as though they were. Do thou likewise.

3. Faith is made perfect by works. Faith always acts accordingly. Faith will go into action after hearing and then believing the truths given by the Lord God about his healing power. Faith that does not act is dead and cannot bring healing. Faith without works is dead being alone. Abraham believed God and acted accordingly by packing up and leaving his home. He had no road map. He had no idea where that land was. But he was looking for a city that had foundation. Only then was his faith counted to him for righteousness. When God told Abraham that he had given him a land to possess, Abraham believed God's statement of fact. Proof that Abraham believed was that he packed up immediately and left his home. By works his faith was perfected or manifest.

Faith means you believe something you cannot prove. Abraham couldn't prove that he possessed a land of milk and honey. But he started walking in that direction anyway, regardless of the weather conditions or the road conditions or the gossip or the hindrances. Regardless of circumstances Abraham obeyed.

HOW YOUR FAITH CAN BRING YOUR HEALING

Set a time and place for your healing. Your time and place is when hands are laid on you or when you speak the words given in this statement of faith in the next section. Then from that point you change what your mouth is saying. You confess what the Word says about you and not what the doctor or your body says about you. Abraham was strong in faith because WHY? Because he considered not his own body. He considered only what the Word of God said about him and not what his body said about him. He believed something he could not prove. He could not prove there was such a land as the Lord had promised. But he believed it enough to stake his life and future on it by packing up and leaving his home.

You have set a time and place for your healing. You are prepared to change what comes out of your mouth. You will confess what the Word says, "By his stripes I am healed" and stop saying what your body or your tests say about your body. Change your confession. Never again say "my cancer". Never again talk about the treatment, the pain, or the circumstances of the past. Only confess what the Word says about you. If you order your speech aright, the Lord promised to show you his salvation.

Then prepare to act accordingly. Get up and walk, stretch forth your hand, do what you could not do before. In some cases people are too weak to stand or walk. But your confession is your action along with what you tell the doctors and your caring ones. I don't want any further treatment until first Medical Science gives me the latest scientific tests from head to toe to determine the true status of my health. And I am getting a second opinion.

Many people are so clearly healed, their tumor disappeared, their pain or discharge stopped immediately. They are so certain of their healing that they immediately tell their doctor and loved ones the following; "Hey doc, thanks for all your treatment. But I have decided to go on a six month vacation. I'll call you if I need you. Don't call me, I'll call you. THEN hang up the phone immediately before some well meaning person talks you out of your healing. And go on that vacation. Get lost. Cancel all appointments. Stop all medication of every kind.

Then get in a church that believes in and teaches and PRACTICES WEEKLY the true Pentecostal power of the Holy Ghost to baptize you and give you a new life and new language and new friends who will encourage you and love you and stand by you

Never disgrace the love of Jesus Christ who healed you body by going back to the sinful blasphemy that teaches that Jesus Christ's power has all passed away and is not for us today. They say that Jesus Christ no longer Baptizes people with the Holy Ghost and has cancelled his promises and cancelled his power for every day miracles to help in time of need. John the Baptist said that Jesus Christ would baptize with the Holy Ghost. Water baptism was John's ministry but Holy Ghost baptism is Jesus Christ's ministry. And he began that ministry on the Day of Pentecost. Don't ever insult the Lord Jesus by listening to or supporting anyone who tells you that Jesus Christ has changed and no longer Baptizes with the Holy Ghost or heals the sick by miracles today. If you do, you give the devil of cancer or affliction legal right to come back into your body with seven more demons worse than him.

Remember, Abraham was strong in faith because he considered not his own body. If you don't consider your own body, then what do you consider? You consider only what the WORD says about your body and not what your body says. That is strong faith and it always performs miracles for the one who observes that path to miracle healing.

FAITH YOU CAN USE RIGHT NOW - - - TO RECEIVE YOUR HEALING

Faith is blind. The Word says we walk by faith and not by sight. Not by sight. Not by sight. Abraham was strong in faith. YOU can have STRONG faith right now just like Abraham had. But why did Abraham have strong faith? Very simple. Because he considered not his own body. His body was powerless, dead, and incapable, past the age of childbearing. But ... He considered NOT his own body. But your doctors have nothing but your body to consider. You consider your body every time your mouth talks your pain, talks your problems, talks your medication, and talks the doctors findings. I know it is difficult for you to stop considering your pains and disease and troubles. But you must become blind to all those things. We walk by faith and not by sight. The things that are seen are temporary, but the things that are NOT SEEN are eternal. Just don't confess your physical feelings.

Stop talking what you feel or see and confess only what the Lord said about your body. Consider the healing Jesus Christ provided for your body. Think on the Word of God and the promises of God for your healing. The Bible commands, THINK ON THESE THINGS. Bring your thoughts into captivity to the obedience of Christ. Think on what God says instead of what your body says. Think on the stripes Jesus took for your healing instead of the medication or treatment your take. If you want strong faith, then stop looking at the physical and natural. Look only at what the Lord says about your body.

Follow these examples and you will be healed.

The woman with the issue of blood said, "If I can but touch the border of his garment I shall be whole." I shall be whole. I shall be whole. If I can but touch the hem of his garment I shall be healed. When you follow the simple instructions in the next section and say what the Word says… you will be healed. Say this right now: **When I say what the Word says about my condition, I will be healed. When I say what the Word says about my condition I will be healed. RIGHT then that minute I will be healed.**

Saying it sows it. Saying it grows it. Saying it knows it. So keep saying it. You will come to believe what your ears hear your mouth saying. Feed yourself faith talk. Talk about what you can't see. Faith lives in the NOT SEEEN world. Faith is the…evidence of things NOT SEEN. Heb 11:1

Notice, that woman wasn't talking about needing money or food or how she hurt or that the doctors took all her money and left her dragging the ground about to die worse than before. No, she fed herself faith talk which looked at what she could not see but wanted to see. Her faith set a time and place for her healing and it worked for her. It will work for you. God is no respecter of persons. Say this, when I make the faith confession and bind the devil of sickness and command it to come out I shall be healed. I won't be sick any more. I shall be healed. I shall be healed.

The blind man with mud on his eyes made with the spit from the mouth of Immanuel was hurrying and bumping and stumbling all the way across town to the pool of Bethesda. For he knew that when he obeyed the instructions of the Word from Jesus he would be healed. When I wash this mud off my eyes, I shall be healed. When I wash this mud off my eyes I shall be healed. When I wash this mud off my eyes I shall be healed. AND IT Worked. And it will work for you just the same.

The last example is the most powerful. A Roman soldier had a servant who was bedridden with sickness nigh unto death. He came to Jesus and spoke his request. Jesus said, I will come and heal him. But the Roman Soldier said, "No Jesus, I am not worth that you come under my roof. But speak the Word only and my servant shall be whole". Speak the Word only and my servant shall be whole.

That Roman soldier set a time and place for the healing of his servant. He said, When Jesus speaks the Word of healing right here right now, then his power will go clear across town to the bed room of my servant and heal my servant. When Jesus speaks the word, my servant shall be whole. When Jesus speaks the word my servant shall be whole. When Jesus speaks the word my servant shall be whole. It worked for that Roman Soldier and it will work for you. Jesus is no respecter of persons.

When you listen to the two part message I will give you about the Cross and the Whipping post; then confess the statement of faith forgiving all your enemies, repenting of all sin, claiming the shed Blood of Jesus as full payment for all your sins, you are ready for healing. If you believe the truth I give about the Cross and the Whipping post then when I call the spirit of sickness out of you it will go instantly and you won't have cancer or AIDS or that affliction from that point on. That is the simple working of the Gift of Healing the Lord bestowed on me during a time of fasting and prayer. Multiplied thousands have been delivered of all manner of sickness and afflictions through this Gift of Healing.

This Gift of Healing worked in Russia, Kenya, East Africa, Canada, Mexico the United States and by phone to many other parts of the world.

Here is a case that will help to build your faith. A family had bought a large estate with a home that had survived the Civil War Era. But the house was cursed with demonic manifestations. Shadows would appear and move around the walls of the rooms. There would be unexplained noises which would sound at various times of the day or night. The entire family was living in fear and planning to move out of the house.

They heard about this ministry and called for help. The family listened to the two part presentation I gave, repented, prayed the statement of faith and then received the Holy Ghost Baptism. They joined in binding the demon spirits and commanding them to go and never return. The first three visits covered teaching the simplicity of the Gospel and their own repentance. Then they learned about the work of demon spirits and the power over the devil that comes with the Baptism of Jesus, called the Baptism of the Holy Ghost. Their religious experience had not included teaching along those lines. The demons manifesting inside the house left the house after the forth visit and never came back. Demons are real and still go about as roaring lions or as angels of light or as ministers of righteousness or whatever it takes to deceive you and torment you.

During the forth visit they all joined in speaking to the demon spirits and binding them in Jesus Name and then commanding them go and never return. Their traditional church never believed or understood what happened. But everyone saw the great change that had taken place in the life of that family.

Please turn to the Apendix pg. 61 and read the amazing faith building testimonies before you proceed.

NOW HERE IT IS: <u>THE TWO PART MESSAGE THE LORD</u>
<u>TOLD ME TO GIVE EVERYONE NEEDING A MIRACLE</u>
<u>HEALING.</u>

PART 1   **NOTE: You must read this carefully.**

THE CROSS AND THE WHIPPING POST

During the long period of fasting and prayer, the Lord Jesus instructed me to tell people two truths from the Word of God. If they will believe these simple statements about the cross and the whipping they would be healed.
The first truth concerns the simplicity of the Gospel; our redemption by the Blood of Jesus Christ. The next truth is that
Jesus took all our sickness into his own body at the whipping post, Matthew 8: 17. 1 Peter 2:24 and Isaiah 53:5

After God created the heavens and the earth, he planted a garden and created a man to live there named Adam. He gave Adam only one commandment, don't eat the fruit of one certain tree, for in the day you eat it you shall surely die. You may eat the fruit from all the other trees but not the fruit of the tree of the knowledge of good and evil.

Then the Lord God made a wife for Adam whom he named Eve. She was tempted by the serpent, satan, to eat the forbidden fruit and she yielded. Then she took the fruit to Adam and he also ate. They were filled with shame due to their nakedness; with guilt because of their sin and with fear because they knew they were under the sentence of death. God hates sin and he promised that the soul that sins shall die. God cannot lie so he had to execute Adam and Eve for their sin.

But God had a big problem. You see he created Adam and Eve. They were in his image and were his own children by creation. He loved them above all other created things. But his problem was that he hates sin. He hates it. He cannot even look upon sin. Not one single sin will ever enter heaven.

However, the Lord loved Adam and Eve too much to strike them the death blow he had promised. But God cannot lie and he is not soft on sin and he must stand behind his word to perform it in every case. So God had a plan. Instead of striking Adam and Eve, he took an innocent snow white lamb and laid it on a stone alter prepared for sacrifice. Then he legally (but not literally) transferred all the sin of Adam and Eve into the very body of that innocent lamb. Next he struck that lamb the death blow which belonged to Adam and Eve. That lamb of God bled and died there in the garden as a substitute for Adam and Eve. The scripture tells us plainly the identity of that lamb. See Rev. 13:8; and 1 Peter 1:18-20.

Then the Lord took the skin of that lamb and made clothing for Adam and Eve and sent them out of the garden. Watch them as they leave that garden. The truth is you can't see Adam and Eve. You see only the snow white clothing of the lamb which was slain as a substitute for them. They look like the lamb. You must see that the Lord made a way to pay for all their sins and remove all the guilt from their hearts for their evil deeds. Adam and Eve contributed nothing what so ever to this plan of redemption. They could offer nothing to help God's plan or improve upon God's plan for redeeming their sinful condition. Jesus paid it all. "And when they had nothing to pay, he forgave them both." Luke 7:42.

God did not deal with, Adam and Eve, according to their sin. He remembered that they were but dust. Ps. 103:10-14. Adam and Eve were accepted in the beloved, Eph. 1:6. Legally they were dead. Paul said, "I am dead to the law of God by the body of Christ" (Gal 2:19). John 3: 16 is known by everyone, For God so loved the world. But you must read the rest of the chapter, for in verse 36 it says that God has wrath upon the world. Wrath and love. Wrath upon the world because he hates sin. Not one sin will ever get by unpunished and the only punishment for any sin is death and eternity in Hell, according to his Word. God hates sin, that's an absolute and eternal truth for all time and all people. So God has wrath against men because of their sin. But at the same time the Lord loves all men and woman. While we were yet sinners Christ died for us. Yes God had a big problem. He loves mankind but hates sin. God's love and hate met together at the Cross on Golgotha's hill.

Now picture in your mind, Jesus hanging on the cross, bloody and beaten, nailed up there, in pain and agony. Jesus took all our sin into his own body on the cross, (1 Peter 2:24). The Lord laid on Jesus the sin of us all, (Is. 53:6). Picture this also in your mind, Jesus was snow white and pure, then suddenly all the sin of mankind was laid within his body. Horrid black, laid on pure white. When the black of man's sins came into the pure white of the Lamb, the sun blacked out, all the universe went dark. The earth shook, and the great mountains split. Matt. 27:51.

Here is where God truly "became" a man. Here is where Jesus earned the title, Son of Man. For he took the sin of all men. And he tasted death for all men. Heb.2:9. But it was our sins appearing in his body that brought down the death blow upon him. It was for me he suffered and bled and died. His death paid for all my sins, past, present and future. 1 Peter 2:24; 2 Cor. 5:21.

FOR GOD TOOK THE SINLESS CHRIST AND POURED INTO HIM OUR SINS. THEN IN EXCHANGE, HE POURED GOD'S GOODNESS INTO US! 2 CORINTHIANS 5:21 (TLB)

The word wrath means boiling anger directed toward an object getting ready to be delivered. The boiling anger was directed toward you and me. But as Jesus hung on the cross and our sins were poured into his innocent body, all the wrath of God was redirected. His wrath turned away from you and me and pointed toward the man on the cross, whose body held all the sins of all the human family from Adam and Eve to the last sin of all time.
Think of it friend. All the sins of all time appeared in one place at one time. In the body of the lamb of God, hanging on that cross. Then God let go his wrath against all our sins and struck the Lamb of God the death blow. His death paid for all our sins for all time, past, present and future. There is no sin except the unpardonable sin, not covered by the Blood of the Lamb shed on Calvary's cross. Your sin debt was marked: PAID IN FULL when Jesus cried his last, "It is finished".

Now the Lord has no wrath against you and me if we come under his Covenant of Blood. Heaven has no more record that you or I ever sinned if we are in CHRIST. Jesus took your record of sins out of your way by nailing it to His cross, Col. 2:13-14. Remember, before those nails pierced his hands, they passed right through your record of sins. His precious life blood has paid for all your sins and your record was blotted out forever. Selah!

Only by the shedding of blood is there remission of sin, Heb 9:22. Nothing can for sin atone, nothing but the blood of Jesus. Not the works of my mind or hand, not money or goodness or good deeds, nothing but the blood of Jesus. For all - that is - ALL - have sinned Jesus said. All except Jesus Christ, so HE ALONE is worthy and could pay for all our sins .

Oh! Precious is the flow that makes me white as snow. No other fount I know- nothing but the blood of Jesus. Jesus loved us and washed us from our sins in his own precious blood, Rev. 1:5. Never trust in a church, or your good works or money given to the church or to the poor or any person's good works. NOTHING BUT THE BLOOD OF JESUS CAN PAY FOR SIN. And all sin was paid for by one stroke of love on the cross of Calvary.

Picture in your mind, Jesus hanging on the cross, beaten, bloody disfigured, nailed to the wood. Now see him hanging there and let me ask you some questions: First, how much did it cost Jesus to get you? Think about it. How much did it cost Jesus to pay for your sin debt?

Next look at Jesus hanging there and tell me, how much does he hate, hate, hate your sins and mine?
Then answer this question, how much are you worth to him? Not in money or possessions. But you... Just you. What is your value? How much are you worth? I found out one day what I am worth. I am worth what it cost to get me. It is sacrifice that creates value, not money. I know how much he loves me and wants me with him, by how much he was willing to pay to get me. Selah!

Part 2

NEXT - YOU MUST SEE THAT JESUS GOT SICK WITH YOUR SICKNESS

"It pleased the Lord to wound him and <u>make him sick</u>."
Isaiah 53:10 (Amp.)

Just before Jesus was nailed to the cross he was whipped and beaten, Matt.27:26. Jesus was so beaten and bloodied, so disfigured, one would scarcely know it was a person standing there, Isa. 52:13-15 (TLB). Pilot laid Jesus' back open with a leaded whip, John 19:1 (TLB). Isa. 53:4. Yet it was our pains he bore, our sickness that weighted him down. He was lashed and we were healed. Yet it was the Lord's good plan to wound him and fill him with sickness, (The Amplified Bible)

Matthew 8: 17 (Jesus) himself, took our sickness and bore our diseases and by his stripes (whipping) we were healed, 1 Peter 2:24. The Hebrew text for Isa. 53:4-5, says, Jesus took wound for wound. For every wound in our bodies, he took a wound in his body. So you see that the healing you want today has already been provided for you. Your name was on one of those stripes. But you must claim it in Jesus Name as Israel had to claim each step of the Promise Land even though it had been given to them before they entered.

"Bless the Lord! Oh my soul and forget not all his benefits; who forgiveth all thine iniquities and healeth all thy diseases." - Ps 103:1-3. Jesus went about doing good - healing all who were oppressed of the devil, Acts 10:38. Not one person Jesus healed was oppressed of god. Matt. 5:18, Jesus said, "My words will never pass away." Those healing words are available to us today for Jesus is the same yesterday, today and forever, Heb. 13:8. Never allow any preacher or other person to tell you that Jesus' miracle healing power has passed away. Jesus said, "I did not come to destroy men's lives but to save them." - Luke 9:56.

SICKNESS COMES FROM SATAN – NOT JESUS

When something very bad happens to us, like having cancer, we usually say, the Lord is on my case. I have been a bad actor and the Lord is punishing me for my sins. But friend, this is not true. Not that you don't have a case. But remember what happened to your case, all your sins were judged on the cross IN CHRIST. Your record of sins were nailed 'to his cross. You are not being punished for your sins. Remember, Heaven has no more record that you ever sinned. You are justified by his precious blood. Selah! It is understood that you must repent of those sins to begin with. Get out of the sin business. It was satan that struck Job with boils, not the Lord. Jesus healed all oppressed of the devil. All sickness is the oppression of the devil, directly or indirectly. Acts 10:38.

Jesus said that he came that we might have life - not cancer, John 10:10. Jesus came to give us all things that pertain to life and godliness, 2 Peter 1:3. Jesus gives love and healing. Then Jesus said, satan came to kill, steal and destroy. Cancer has Satan's fingerprints all over it. It is Satan that brought this cancer or disease on you and not the Lord Jesus. Jesus came to destroy the works of the devil, and he succeeded, 1 John 3:8. Cancer is Satan's work. I want to lift this cancer off your soul and put it on Jesus where it belongs. It is his cancer. He took it because he loves you. Jesus is your High Priest and is touched, touched with the feelings of your body; the feelings of your infirmities. Heb. 4: 15.

NOW! IF YOU CAN SEE YOUR SICKNESS APPEARING IN HIS BODY YOU ARE <u>STANDING ON HEALING GROUND</u>!

Last of all, picture in your mind, the body of Jesus hanging on that whipping post being beaten with the whips. Now see your sickness and pain appearing in his body. That is when Jesus took our sickness and bore our diseases. Matt. 8:17. That's when Jesus took, **"WOUND FOR WOUND". FOR EACH WOUND IN OUR BODIES, A WOUND APPEARED IN THE BODY OF CHRIST AS HE WAS WHIPPED, Isa 53:5.**

NOTICE: THE VERY SICKNESS AND PAIN IN YOUR BODY RIGHT NOW HAS ALREADY BEEN ON THIS EARTH ONCE BEFORE – 2000 YEARS AGO IT APPEARED IN THAT BODY HANDING ON THAT WHIPPING POST!

That means that your sickness has already appeared on the earth once before. It appeared in the body of that man tied to the whipping post nearly 2,000 years ago. Now, see your sickness appearing in his body, for the Word says, Jesus TOOK our sickness and BORE our infirmities. Matt. 8:17. The word 'took' is a legal term which means TITLE PASSED. The title to your sickness actually passed to Jesus the Lamb of God, for in his loving plan for you he legally TOOK your sickness into his own body.

That means that whatever sickness or cancer you may have doesn't legally belong to you anymore. Jesus took it. Selah! WHY? Because he loves you and doesn't want you to have it. "I will take sickness away from (you)." Ex. 23:55.

As Moses lifted up the serpent in the wilderness, even so must the Son of Man be lifted up…. John 3:14. Looking at that serpent brought healing for their physical affliction. We have a better covenant. Healing is by the stripes Jesus took on his body.

That serpent is what we (in our sins) looked like to the Father. But as many as LOOKED received healing in their bodies. Look at Jesus hanging on the whipping post with your sickness in his body, for he took your sickness. See Jesus hanging on the cross with all your sins poured into his body, for he took our sins on the Cross. If you can see your sickness and pain appearing in the Body of Christ during his whipping, you are ready to be healed. Close your eyes and SEE Jesus filled with your pain and sickness.

Contact me for immediate help and prayer. See pg 87 for contact info

SAY THIS PRAYER OUT LOUD WITH ALL YOUR OWN HEART

Lord Jesus, I thank you for the blood you shed on the Cross for my sins. It was my sins appearing in your body that brought down the death blow upon you. That means you died for me. I love you for that Jesus. I worship you for that Jesus. Now I repent of all my sins. I am truly sorry for all my sins. I renounce the sins of my ancestors. I break every family curse and every witchcraft curse pronounced against me. I forgive all my enemies. I forgive everyone who has ever hurt me. I open my heart and let them go. Come into my heart and fill me with the Holy Ghost.
 Forgive me Jesus. Wash me in the Blood of your Cross and I will be pure and clean from all my sins, Rev. I:5.

NOW CONTINUE READING OUT LOUD FROM YOUR HEART

It is written, Jesus took all my sickness into his own body. So I don't want it back. I don't have to have it. I now withdraw permission for cancer to work in my body. You devil of fear and doubt. You devil of cancer. I bind you in Jesus Name and command you to come out of my body. Go in Jesus name and never come back. I plead the Blood of Jesus over my soul and body. Devil you can't cross the Blood of Jesus to ever come back. I now confess, the Blood of Jesus Christ paid for all my sins and by his stripes I am healed. I worship you Jesus. I love you Jesus. Thank you for healing my body of all sickness and disease.

You are healed if you really believed the Word of the Lord. Multitudes have been healed through confessing the words of this book. You too can be healed through obeying the instructions in this book. But I will minister to you personally if you will contact me.

NEXT, VALIDATE YOUR HEALING

Now turn to someone near you or call them on the phone and confess this Bible verse to them, "By His stripes I am healed", I Peter

2:24. Say it over and over. Notice that when you say that verse, it challenges your own faith.

Then confess the My Daily Confession Sheet on Pg.85, twice a day for 21 days. It will transform your life.
Keep testifying that Bible Verse, "By His stripes I AM HEALED". You will never rise above your confession. You will never possess until you first confess. Romans 10:8-10, says that only if we CONFESS, will we then POSSESS. Keep confessing your healing and thank the Lord Jesus right now and many times daily for your healing. Faith means, you believe something you cannot prove. You now walk by faith and not by sight.

THE CANCER DEVIL LEFT YOUR BODY if you believed the Word of the Lord. How do I know for sure? Because the Gift of Healing works by speaking to the devil instead of praying. When I speak to that devil and bind it in Jesus Name it HAS TO GO. AND that cancer devil left your body when you spoke to it in Jesus Name, if you believed the Word of the Lord. Now keep it out by confessing the Lord's word. That is VALIDATING your healing. Contact me immediately and I will minister personally to you by phone if necessary. Thousands have been healed that way.

Don't let your loved ones or medical personnel talk you out of your healing. For the first few days you will feel some nausea because your body is throwing off the residue of strong chemicals and decaying cancer cells. This is a sign that you have been healed.

REMEMBER: YOUR HEALING MIRACLE IS NEVER COMPLETE - - - UNTIL YOU TESTIFY THAT YOU ARE HEALED. Your testimony completes your healing. Your testimony validates your healing. Saying it sows it. So say it.
WARNING!   You must never go back into the religion that failed to bring you healing! Read again the case of Naaman the leper, pg. 9, who changed his religion to worship the God that healed him.

ALSO: YOUR DOCTOR DOESN'T KNOW YOU HAVE BEEN HEALED

So he will want to continue to treat you as usual. If you let this happen, you are in serious trouble. If you continue his treatment without a word, **you are denying your healing**.

VERY IMPORTANT- - - Tell your doctor that you want him to give you the latest scientific examination before he does anything else to you. And tell him you are getting a second opinion. THIS IS A MUST! He will not like that but you are the one fighting for your life against cancer or other diseases, not him. Insist against his objections all of which are invalid and non-binding.

Most people, when healed by Jesus of cancer, are so blest, there is no question about their healing. Everyone can see it. But in many cases the healing doesn't appear outwardly enough to satisfy the unbelieving.
Don't play games with the Word of the Lord or with your life. A person who doesn't have cancer should never receive any cancer treatment

In some cases when your doctor sees that your cancer is gone he will say it is in remission. Remission means that the cancer is not 'healed' but only lurking out of sight within your body ready to strike again at any time.

You are the one that has been fighting death, not your doctor or your husband or your wife or loved ones or family or friends. You and you alone must make the decisions affecting your medical care. THEREFORE: Tell your doctor that you don't want him to treat you in any way until he has checked you by two of the latest scientific methods to determine the status of your health. Also, be VERY SURE to tell your doctor you are going to get a second opinion.

When your doctor checks you over, he will likely say one of two things:

a) You are much better; the cancer is all gone except a little up here or down there ... etc. etc. So that proves my treatment is working. Now take just 6 or 8 more shots of chemotherapy so that the cancer won't come back.

If you let him do this without a second opinion you are in trouble. Call me first and I will minister again to you if there is any valid reason to do so.   I have found that many doctors will not tell their cancer patients the whole truth for fear of malpractice suites. **GET A** **SECOND OPINION**.

If you accept the doctor's statement and allow him to give you further cancer treatment, you give the cancer devils legal right to return. Call me immediately and I will minister to you again if you feel the need for it.

b) Or your doctor might say, "the cancer is gone."   This proves my treatment is working. He will take all the credit for your improvement. Now you must take 6 or 8 more shots of chemotherapy (or other cancer treatment) to keep the cancer from coming back. DON'T DO IT. Doctors do not believe in miracle healings. They could make no money that way.

Again, if you accept this statement from the doctor and receive his treatment, you are denying the healing power you received from the Lord Jesus.

More important yet: You must never go back into the church that failed to bring you healing. I will help you find a true Pentecostal type church.

Jesus clearly said in John 5: 14, that when a person is healed of a physical infirmity, if they go back into (sin) their former way of life, the infirmity will come back upon them in a worse form. Read it for yourself. Also in Matt. 12:43-45, Jesus said that when a demon spirit is cast out of a person, it will go seeking rest, and will try to come back into the person it came out of. And if that person's life is empty of the things of the Spirit and praises of the Lord, the demon will get 7 more demons worse than itself and re-enter that person and the last state of that man is worse than the first.

A church or minister who says Jesus stopped his ministry of Gifts and Holy Ghost Baptism is lying on Jesus. It is a mortal sin to listen to or support a ministry like that. Jesus said, if a church denies the POWER, get out of there. Don't listen to them.

SO? Get the complete latest scientific examination and also a second opinion and you will feel safe about any decision you then make.

GOOD NEWS! At least 80% of all cancer victims who have been healed by the power of God, manifest their healing in such a way that they and everyone around them can see it and just don't doubt their miracle healing. For example, tumors disappear; sick feelings and fever or swelling goes immediately.

Contact me for immediate help and prayer. See pg 87 for contact info

<u>IF FEAR, DOUBT OR A SYMPTOMS SHOW UP - PLACE YOUR HAND OVER JESUS' NAME</u>

AND CONFESS ALOUD THE FAITH STATEMENT BELOW.

Say it out loud – very loudly!

THE LORD JESUS CHRIST

Speak at the top of your voice….shout it out….say this confession now…

IN THE NAME OF JESUS CHRIST, I'M NOT AFRAID OF YOU SATAN. I COMMAND YOU DEVIL OF FEAR AND DOUBT, YOU DEVIL OF CANCER AND AFFLICTION COME OUT OF MY BODY. I withdraw permission for you to work in my body. It is written: Jesus took my sickness so I don't have to have it. I don't want it any longer.

I CALL THE BLOOD OF JESUS CHRIST OVER MY SOUL AND BODY. SATAN YOU CANNOT CROSS THE BLOOD. YOU CANNOT RETURN. I AM COVERED BY THE BLOOD OF JESUS CHRIST. I NOW CONFESS, BY THE WOUNDS OF JESUS, I AM HEALED.

Repeat this statement several times out loud. You will experience the power of a renewed faith and assurance of your healing. You won't have to do this but a few times and the fear or FALSE symptoms will never return.

FIRST get into a church that teaches what I teach. This ministry of the Gift of Healing brought you a miracle. Worship the God that brought you healing. Read 2 Kings Chapter 5. When the leper was healed, he left his church and worshipped the God that answered by fire, the God that healed him. It would have been like mockery to go back to the god that failed to save his life and bring his miracle healing. Call or write me, I can help you find a church like you need. Serve the God that answers by fire. Never go back to the church that failed to bring you a life saving miracle or that denies miracles and the Holy Ghost Baptism as in Acts 2:4.

It is a blasphemy to teach a lie about Jesus Christ, that he quit Baptizing with the Holy Ghost and quit healing the sick.
THE LORD JESUS SAID: These signs shall follow them that believe, …they shall cast out devils.
HE also said, "The 12 went everywhere preaching the word and the Lord went with them, working miracles on the sick and diseased, to show that he approved of the message that they preached." Mark 16:20. Listen to the scriptures. You will be blest.

EXAMPLE: A doctor (DC) took me to a 12 month old baby boy with liver cancer which grew from its liver to 3 inches out the front of its body. I ministered the Word to the parents and then laid hands on the baby and the cancer devil came out instantly. The very next day, when the doctor saw the child he recognized that the cancer was dead and that the child's kidneys which had been totally destroyed by chemo therapy were working again. The doctor knew this at first glance. So there was no question that the child didn't need any further medical treatment. But some cases are not so obvious so follow these instructions and you will be safe.

Another case: Pam Ross a lady priest of the Anglican church of Canada had cancer. Two large tumors protruded from her left side and abdomen. She had only days to live. I gave the words and she prayed the sinner's prayer. When I lifted my hands from her head with the words, "Come out," She grabbed her left side and said that thing is gone. The tumors disappeared instantly. She had been on baby food for three months but could immediately eat a cheese burger prepared for her. Her healing was so obvious that there was never any question in her mind or the mind of anyone who knew her that she didn't need further medical treatment.

Bertha Scott at the Med Center, Memphis TN, was given up to die. The doctors called the family in one day saying Bertha would not live through the night. She had bone cancer in the left leg just above her knee and just below her hip joint. I got there in the afternoon before the family gathered. I ministered to Bertha, who had been a member of my church many years before. She believed and the cancer devil came out instantly. All pain and throbbing left her instantly. She slept through the night for the first time in months. The next morning she awoke feeling find and asked for scrambled eggs and toast. The family was distraught and called the doctor in and angrily questioned him about his warning. The doctors were fearful of malpractice so they said they would have to examine her to be sure what happened. The x-rays and all tests clearly showed cancer in the last stages. That was 5 years ago. Today Bertha is still healthy and strong and 82 years of age getting around like a middle age woman. Glory!

PART 3

GO AND SHOW YOURSELF

FOR A TESTIMONY - - Not to SEE **if** you are really healed!

Your testimony completes your healing. In Matt. 9:21, the woman with the issue of blood said ... "If I may but touch the border of his garment, I shall be whole." She touched his garment and immediately she received her healing. She fed herself faith script. She confessed her healing instead of her sickness. Do thou likewise.

But notice, Jesus asked "Who touched me?", and kept asking till the woman testified to her healing. Then AND ONLY THEN did Jesus said to her, "Daughter, thy faith has made thee whole". Her public testimony validated her healing.

She had to testify to her healing before Jesus pronounced her made whole. You must tell someone immediately that, "By his stripes, I am healed". Testify now.

Note: The greatest mistake you can make is to wait for the doctor to tell you the cancer is gone. You must exercise your faith now and testify to your healing. The Word says you are healed. Say what the Word says about your body and not what your body says. Agree with the Word by confessing it. Call me as quickly as you can get to a phone and let me help you at this critical point.

The ten lepers were told to go show themselves to the priests. As they went they were healed. Only one came back to testify to the Lord and thereby confess his healing and thank the Lord for his healing from leprosy. Then Jesus said to this one, "Arise, go thy way: thy faith has made thee whole", Luke 17:19. Only the leper who testified and gave the Lord Jesus thanks and glory for his healing, completed his healing and was made whole.

Here is your duty, "Let the redeemed of the Lord say so, whom he has redeemed from the hand of the enemy," Ps. 107:2. Give thanks unto the Lord and make known his deeds among the people. Talk of his wondrous works. 1 Chronicles 16:8.

To testify that Jesus Christ has healed you, increases your faith and validates your healing. Jesus will do his part and heal you, but you alone can validate your healing by your confession and testimony that Jesus has healed you. If you don't "go and show", meaning to testify to your healing you may lose your healing. Luke 17:19, "Go and show yourselves .... for a testimony". NOT TO SEE if you are healed but to testify that you are healed. Notice the difference and obey it.

CAN SICKNESS COME BACK ON A PERSON?
Very Definitely!

In John 5:1-18, Jesus healed a man at the pool of Bethesda.

Later that day, vs. 14, Jesus found the man and told him if he went back into his former way of life, this sickness would come back on him in a worse form. Yes! Sickness can and does come back on people if they don't live a life which honors the Lord Jesus who is the Healer. Out of love and thanksgiving and honor for your healer, Jesus Christ, you must praise his name and testify about your healing. If you refuse to do so, it could open the door to Satan to strike you again with a worse condition. It is blasphemy to say that Jesus no longer Baptizes with the Holy Ghost or heals through the Gifts of the Spirit. It is a sin and if you go back into that kind of religion, you give satan legal right to strike again.

CAN DEVILS RE-ENTER A PERSON?

Once cast out, can demon spirits return to a body which they formally inhabited? Yes they can. In Matt. 12:43, Jesus said, "When the unclean spirit (all demons are unclean) is gone out of a man, he walketh through dry places seeking rest, and findeth none. Then the spirit says, I will return to my house whence I came out: and when he is come, he findeth it empty, swept and garnished. Then goeth he, and taketh with himself 7 other spirits more wicked than himself, and they enter in and dwell there: and the last state of that man is worse than the first". Yes! Once cast out, a demon spirit can re-enter the same person again, but notice why the demon can enter.

If your house (body) is empty, swept and garnished, you automatically give the demon spirit a legal right to re-enter your body and bring seven more demons with him. Your last illness will be 7 times worse than your first. By disobeying the Lord and refusing to testify the demon has a legal right to torment you.

LIKE NAAMAN THE SYRIAN – leave the church that couldn't bring you healing and join the one that did bring you healing like a true Pentecostal Church and worship the God that answered by fire and healed you. Find one and attend from this day.

Don't leave your life empty. Fill your life with the Baptism of the Holy Ghost and with the study of the Word of God and attending a church that preaches and teaches the truth of the Word about miracles and healings. If you go back to a church which denies miracles-- you sin against the one who healed you. You will lose faith and get sick again. If you support a ministry that fights the Bible truth of miracles for today and the power of the Holy Ghost today you are asking for trouble. You will lose your faith and lose your healing. You will have dishonored the Lord Jesus who healed you. You will thereby give demon spirits a legal right to re-enter your life and torment you much worse than before.

GOOD NEWS!   YOU DON'T HAVE TO ACCEPT SICKNESS AND PAIN WHEN IT COMES

NOTE THIS GREAT TRUTH: "RESIST THE DEVIL AND HE WILL FLEE FROM YOU." JAMES 4:7.

Sickness and pain originates with the devil and demon spirits. Notice that Jesus cast out, deaf spirits, dumb spirits, blind spirits, insane spirits and many different kinds of spirits, indicating that demon spirits were causing the physical afflictions and pain.

"So went Satan forth from the presence of the LORD, and smote Job with sore boils from the sole of his foot unto his crown." (Job 2:7 KJV).   The devil struck Job with boils.

"And, behold, there was a woman which had a spirit of infirmity eighteen years, and was bowed together, and could in no wise lift up herself."
"And when Jesus saw her, he called her to him, and said unto her, Woman, thou art loosed from thine infirmity."
"And he laid his hands on her: and immediately she was made straight, and glorified God."

"And ought not this woman, being a daughter of Abraham, whom Satan hath bound, lo, these eighteen years, be loosed from this bond on the Sabbath day?"

"And when he had said these things, all his adversaries were ashamed:

and all the people rejoiced for all the glorious things that were done by him." (Luke 13:11-17 KJV)

It was Satan that bound that poor woman for 18 years.

"And, behold, a woman of Canaan came out of the same coasts, and cried unto him, saying, Have mercy on me, O Lord, thou son of David; my daughter is grievously vexed with a devil." (Mat 15:22 KJV)

A spirit of infirmity from the devil was afflicting this child and Jesus cast out the devil and the child was healed.

Further proof is from Acts 10:38 "Jesus went about doing good... healing all who were oppressed of the devil." All sickness is oppression of the devil, even when no demon spirit is present. Jesus has given power over the devil. It is true that not every sickness or affliction is caused by the presence of a demon spirit. But healing applies to these cases also, for Jesus heals the sick no matter what the root cause.

Remember also, that medical science has never 'seen' a demon spirit. Doctor's can't see demons through their instruments like X-Rays and other testing equipment.

And one of the blessings of being a Holy Ghost filled Christian is, you have power over the devil. Jesus said, "these signs shall follow them that believe, in My Name...they shall cast out devils." Mark 16:17.

First Jesus gave the 12 disciples power over the devil. In Luke 9: "I give you power over all the power of the devil." Matthew 10: "I give you power over all the power of the devil." Then in Luke 10, Jesus called 70 more men and sent them out two by two and said, "I give you power over all the power of the devil." That made 82 men going around casting out devils in Jesus Name. They all returned to Jesus rejoicing that devils were subject to them through Jesus Name.

Remember also, that Jesus took your sickness when they whipped him. He took all sickness. So you don't have to have it. Quote that verse to the devil and he will have to retreat immediately. When pain or sickness strikes you, you don't have to receive it. You can bind the pain or sickness and command it to come out of your body in the Name of Jesus Christ and it will have to go.

I well remember the first time a severe pain struck my body on my left side just below my ribs. It was so severe I doubled up and almost blacked out. My first thought was that it was an attack of the devil. I immediately spoke to the pain and bound it in Jesus Name and commanded it to come of my body. Immediately the pain eased up and left as suddenly as it had come.

Even medical science says that a person cannot get cancer without their permission. Doctors recognize that people invite sickness sometimes. When someone has been abandoned by a loved one or been betrayed by their spouse, they feel devalued and worthless and unloved and unwanted. That is when they allow or 'invite' sickness to come into their bodies. Your own will plays a part in your sickness. You don't have to accept pain or sickness.

WHY DO SOME PEOPLE INVITE SICKNESS OR WELCOME PAIN AND AFFLICTION?

Why would anyone invite sickness? When they have failed in life or feel they cannot compete on the same level as others and they need an excuse for their failures, they invite pain and sickness. They 'use' that pain and sickness or affliction as their legitimate excuse for failing to 'keep up' with the pack. Their disability then becomes their claim to normalcy and respectability. They have a legitimate excuse for not 'measuring up' to expectations or performing as the average person is expected to perform.

This also explains one of the reasons why some people just never get 'healed' no matter how much medical treatment they receive or how much prayer is expended on their behalf. They hold on to the affliction. They fear facing the world without their 'crutch'. Love covers a multitude of sin and also heals the soul and mind of the many scars of past insults and failures and defeats.

But what about the case where there is something like an organic malfunction like the presence of a growth or a clot blocking an artery or an enflamed body part, or when some bodily functions shuts down and your life is at risk. Still, pain or some physical symptom will alert you to the problem and you can still lay your hand over the pain or over your heart and you can repeat the statement,

"NO DEVIL, NOT ME. IT IS WRITTEN, JESUS CHRIST TOOK MY SICKNESS AND BORE MY DISEASES, AND I DON'T WANT THIS PAIN OR SICKNESS. I DON'T' HAVE TO HAVE IT. I BIND YOU DEVIL OF AFFLICTION AND PAIN AND COMMAND YOU IN THE NAME OF JESUS CHRIST TO COME OUT OF MY BODY."

Then, throw your hand out away from your body to point the pathway for the retreating defeated demon spirit of affliction and pain. Do this with all your heart. If you don't feel complete relief the first time, do it again and again. Remember, no devil can resist a command given in the Name of Jesus Christ. That is impossible and cannot happen. If you say the above confession the pain or clot or blockage or growth will go in Jesus Name.

However you must first read this book and my book on Faith to prepare on this subject and prepare your faith to fight the good fight of faith. You see, faith is a fight. It doesn't take super faith but it does take faith. And faith comes from hearing the Word of God.

Read the two books and be ready to help others who are sick or afflicted. Then your faith will be strong enough to sustain your health in time of peril or plague. The more you exercise your faith the stronger your faith grows.

PART 4

THE URGENT NEED FOR FOOD SUPPLEMENTS

Cancer must live from the food carried in your blood stream just like you do. Therefore cancer drains the life giving nutrients from your blood and other organs of your body. But chemotherapy does much worse than cancer. The goal of chemotherapy is, in effect, to turn your blood almost to water, so as to deny the cancer its food supply. That is why a person who has taken chemotherapy feels so weak and lifeless and their hair falls out. Chemotherapy does the same thing to a human body that AID'S does. It destroys all the body's immune system, which fights diseases, as well as all the anti-bodies created by childhood vaccinations. This leaves the cancer victim open to any germ that may come along.

Radiation treatment is even worse. It fries the human body just like cooking meat in an overheated skillet. The goal is to kill the diseased tissue, but it also kills the healthy tissue in the area of the disease. It's like shooting the side of a wooden barn with a double barreled shotgun hoping to kill the worms eating the wood. Many doctors admit that medical scientists are only experimenting with most cancer patients who receive radiation or chemotherapy. More patients die from radiation sickness or chemo therapy than from cancer.

NOTE: It is very difficult to ever fully recover from radiation sickness. This is why most death certificates of cancer victims do not list the 'cause of death' as cancer but some other disease. Radiation treatment now guarantees that the cancer will come back due to the radiation treatment. Radiation can cause cancer.

ONCE YOU HAVE BEEN HEALED BY THE POWER OF THE LORD JESUS CHRIST - - -

You must act quickly to rebuild your immune system and your entire body. Taking food supplements and vitamins is the only way to do this. Food supplements are not chemicals, drugs or medicines. They are food - highly concentrated food. I urge each one that has been healed of cancer to begin immediately to take the following food supplements which can be found at any health food store.

I. Take Kyo-Green daily, two heaping teaspoons. There is nothing on the market to compare with this product. I have searched for years and found none better. You can order it for less than half what Health Food Stores charge. Ask for the address.

2. Liver tablets. Get a good name brand desiccated liver. Take as directed.

3. Take Bee Pollen, about one to two teaspoons daily. Do not use the tablet form. The capsule form is acceptable if you cannot find the bulk granule form. It is not difficult to find the golden grains of pollen in bulk form.

4. Take a quality one-a-day Vitamin-Mineral, Supplement. Ask your Health Food store to recommend a quality product.

5. Eat low fat yogurt daily. Mix with grape juice or other juices if you desire.

6. Take Pycnogenol daily. This is very important. Grape seed extract is a good substitute for pycnogenol and may be less expensive.

7. Take Allicin Rich Garlic. There are many brands. Get 100% pure Garlic which is Allicin Rich. Fresh garlic is far better.

8. Take Vitamin C daily. About 5000 milligrams total per day of Ester-C. You could take one tablet per hour until you have taken the 5000 milligrams. Dr. Pauling recommends a larger dose.

9. Take Bone Builder Calcium like Citracal.

10. Daily take ¾ cup warm water, mix in one tablespoon raw Honey and stir. Then stir in 2 tablespoons of raw unpasteurized Apple Cider Vinegar and drink in sips. NOTE: Use only raw honey if possible.

11. Take Sublingual B-12 in liquid or tablet form and follow directions for daily intake.

12. Begin drinking Distilled Water Only. Drink at least 8 glasses daily. Drinking ½ gallon daily for the first week is recommended.

13. Eat all the Raw Fruits and Vegetables you can. Or you may use a quality juicer and drink the juice daily. Frozen fruits are now available. Put them in a blender if possible and mix juices to taste.

14. Take Vitamin E daily.

EXERCISE - - You have no choice! You MUST exercise! No matter how weak you may feel you can exercise.

Hold your shoes, one in each hand, and raise your arms up and down till you feel tired. Do this several times daily. Try it with a #2 or #3 can of vegetables in each hand, then something heavier. Put on your shoes and lift your legs as high as you can. Do this several times daily. Do sit-ups as much as you can daily. Exercise is vital to regaining your physical health. Walking is a must, if only around your room or house.

THE FAMILY MUST PARTICIPATE IN THE HEALING – BY THEIR LOVING SUPPORT

Remember the little girl of 12 who died after a long sickness. Jesus raised her from the dead. He gave her back her life minus the sickness. But then Jesus turned to the parents and said, "Give her something to eat." The great miracle wrought on the little girl, didn't include putting flesh and muscle back on her emaciated frame. **The caregivers were called upon to participate in that miracle and keep it going until full physical health was restored**. Taking good food in the form of food supplements is the best way to obey Jesus' command today, "Give them to eat." If you can't take the recommended amounts start with small portions and work up. If you feel nauseated by any of the products, practice tasting the product for several days or try to mix the product with a liquid and sip slowly.

BUT - WHEN YOUR BEST EFFORTS FAIL

There are times when some people will not be healed no matter how we try and cry and travail and pray. Our best efforts sometimes fail. Guilt is often the handmaiden of grief. So is bitterness. We must remember that as humans even the best of us are still looking through the dark side of the glass no matter how great our faith (1 Cor. 12:10-13). We still say of Jesus, "Whom having not seen, we love," I Peter 1:8

Nothing ever comes into our lives, until it first passes through the love of God. Think about that. Selah! To be absent from the body is to be present with the Lord, 2Cor. 5:8. Jesus said to one man, Today, you shall be with me in Paradise," Luke 23:43. When the beggar died, a company of angels was standing by and immediately carried the beggar to Heaven and peace and plenty and comfort forever, Luke 16:22.

Death is not the opposite of life. Jesus taught that dying was a part of life; a move from one level of existence to a higher level of existence. Dying is not the defeat of life; it is a release into the beginning of eternal life with Jesus Christ our Lord.

Dying is not the failure of faith. It is appointed unto man once to die', Heb. 9:27. This is God's immutable law. The Gift of Healing was not given to repeal that law but only as a temporary stay at best. "O! Death, where is thy sting? O! Grave, where is thy victory?" Comfort one another with these words. Both death and the grave have been defeated in that battle which Jesus won for each of us, atop Golgotha's hill and by that empty tomb in the garden.

If you see your loved one approaching the end of life, don't try to hold them or make them more stressful with your begging or pleading for them not to go. You must perform your last noble act for your loved one and crown their life with the honor and dignity it deserves. Give them permission to die. It has been said that most terminally ill patients die in the wee hours of the morning between midnight and six a.m.

when the caregivers are resting or dozing, and the family is asleep. They depart in quietness and peace. We must let them go to a better existence, a better world, where the peace of God reigns.

After my daughter Patricia died of cancer, one of her friends had a dream about her. And in that dream Patricia was seen in a white robe and smiling. When asked, "Patricia, have you seen Jesus yet?" she replied, "I've not only seen Him, I've eaten with him." I weep for joy every time I think of that. To be absent from the body is to be present with the Lord. Comfort one another with these words.

Bless your last moments together by remembering the good times. Be sure you tell them that you commend them to the grace and love of Jesus, the loving Shepherd of their soul. Read them John 14:1-4. Tell them Jesus is coming to escort them to their new home.

One more thing... Don't blame yourself. Death causes each of us to face the stark reality of our own helplessness in the face of the unknown where we must walk alone. Whosoever shall call on the Name of the Lord shall be delivered. Call on the name of Jesus. One of his names is Comforter, and another, the Bishop of our Souls. He will escort your loved one forever more, beginning with their last breath.

Sorrow is a wound. Sorrow is a deep wound. But sorrow is a clean wound. It will heal nicely if no dirt or grit gets in there; like bitterness or self-blame or grief or regret.

Please contact the author for prayer or to order written material, you may write or call:

Rev. Robert L. Bufkin, PO Box 17382; Jonesboro AR 72403. Or call 206-203-6273.

VISIT my web site: http://www.rlbm.org   Send an email: anelijah@fastmail.fm Order the FREE books listed on the website.

NOTICE: Reading the testimonies in the Appendix will greatly strengthen your faith. Please read them carefully.

APPENDIX

These miracles are written that you might believe that Jesus Christ is the Son of the Living God and that Jesus is still alive and still works miracles of salvation and healing. John 20:30-31.

MAKE KNOWN HIS DEEDS AMONG THE PEOPLE

Case # 1

A man named Nobe had been an alcoholic most of his life, had not drawn a sober breath for 7 years, had cancer of the liver, his chest was so full of cancer, his lungs would not show on the X-Ray. His abdomen and mid-section were so filled with cancer, the doctor said it looked like bouquets of flowers pushed into his body. He was in the hospital and given 2 days to live. Fifty-two quarts of fluid had been drawn off his body in three days.

A relative invited me to minister to him one Sunday afternoon at 4:30 p.m. As I entered the room, Nobe testified later that he saw a light covering me and I stepped out of that light and stood beside his bed. I began to give him the words the Lord Jesus told me to say. Then I spoke to the cancer and the devils came out instantly.

The power of the Holy Ghost fell on Nobe and he spoke in an unknown language for several minutes. He was completely healed instantly. I had not mentioned the Baptism of the Holy Ghost to Nobe. The Lord did it.

His doctors examined him closely on Monday for several hours and could find no sign of any cancer in his body. The nodules of cancer were gone from his liver, all the cancer was gone from his body and from within his lungs and chest. Nobe was dismissed from the hospital on Thursday. His doctors angrily refused to allow Nobe to tell them that he had a miracle. They were not only puzzled but also shocked at the sudden and total disappearance of all cancer from his body, and all his healing of all disease. He was also healed of a lifetime of alcoholism, diabetes and Pancreatic cancer. That was in April 1990.

The instant change in Nobe's character was as much of a shock to the entire city where he lived, as was his miraculous healing of cancer. This is the greatest healing I have ever seen in Northeast Mississippi. It truly shook the entire area. All protestants fought it and denied it and gloated with he died ten years later.

Case # 2

A 10-month-old baby boy named Daniel Hinds. Cancer had replaced his spinal cord. Daniel had no control over his extremities. His eyes, head and arms moved liked the limbs of a lifeless doll. Doctors said that there was no treatment possible and that Daniel could die at any time. A businessman brought Daniel to my healing services in Memphis, TN. I touched his right foot and spoke the words of healing. The cancer devils came out immediately. Daniel's mother took him to the doctors two days later. After two hours of intensive examination the doctors reported to the mother these exact words, "The cancer is not active." The doctors refused to give Jesus Christ the praise and glory for the healing miracle. Within a few weeks the large black growth, which had covered his backbone area, was gone. That was in 1989. Today Daniel is a healthy, intelligent little boy showing no signs that he ever had a life threatening cancer.

Case # 3

A nurse who had breast cancer which had spread to another part of her body - her name is Geraldine. She was scheduled for surgery for Wednesday, but asked me to minister to her on the previous Sunday. I gave her the words the Lord instructed me to say. I called the devil of cancer out in Jesus Name and it left instantly. On Wednesday the doctors could find no cancer but insisted on doing a biopsy. Geraldine was free of cancer. No surgery was done. That was in 1991. Today, (in 2000), Geraldine is still praising the Lord for her healing.

Case # 4

Mrs. Mildred J. had cancer and received surgery. But the cancer came back and she received a colostomy. She heard about this Gift of

Healing and drove to my home in 1994 for ministry. She received the words about the Cross and Whipping Post. I spoke the healing words, commanded the cancer devils to come out and they left. Immediately the Holy Ghost fell on her and she spoke in other tongues. After several weeks of examination, showing that Mildred was free of cancer, the doctors reversed her colostomy. This was the first time in the history of that hospital at Water Valley MS that a colostomy had been reversed. In 1995, Mildred, is still healed and praising the Lord for her miracle.

Case # 5

Mrs. Griffin. She taught Spanish at Memphis TN high school. She had cancer surgery in the 1980's but the cancer came back in a different and more dangerous form in 1989. She came to my meeting in June of 1990, and came forward for ministry. I spoke the healing words, called the devil out, laid my hands on her and she fell backward on the floor. She spoke in a new language as she fell. Also, Mrs. Griffin testified later that while falling, before her body hit the floor, she felt all the tumors go from her body. She was a schoolteacher and had already prepared for death. She went back to teaching school in Memphis TN.

Case # 6

Ray, a Baptist, chartered an airplane and flew to another state to meet me and receive the ministry of the Gift of Healing. Doctors had done surgery for one cancer but he refused surgery on the other cancer. He was frightened but willing to exercise faith. The cancer devil came out instantly. Two days later the doctors could not believe that the cancer was gone. Five biopsies showed no cancer in his body.

Case # 7

Rev. Otis, a Baptist preacher, had cancer of the brain and lymph glands of the neck. He had received brain surgery, chemical therapy and radiation but the cancer was advancing rapidly. He heard about this gift and came to a meeting and received ministry. The cancer devils came out instantly and he was filled with the Holy Ghost and spoke in other tongues as the Spirit gave him utterance. Otis' doctors were shocked that suddenly he had no sign of cancer in his body, however, they insisted on continuing chemotherapy, saying that the cancer was only in remission and could come back at any time. The doctors refused to give Jesus Christ praise for a healing miracle. For over a year and a half, Otis received regular check-ups and tests and was consistently pronounced free of all cancer by his doctors. That was in 1990. In 1992, he died of complications of so much radiation and chemical therapy. His wife announced that he did not die of cancer. He had over 18 months of life, free of cancer.

Case # 8

AIDS victim - Mr. DB. A professional, married with 3 children, a bi-sexual. Five years after Mr. DB was diagnosed as having the HIV virus, symptoms began to tell his closely guarded secret. He wife persuaded him to come to me for ministry. It took two hours for him to see the Roman's Road to salvation and that Jesus would never skip over the voluntary devil - sodomy, to heal his involuntary devil of A.I.D.S. He finally repented. Then I had him repeat out loud his repentance of sin and call the devil of lust out of his body. I then spoke to the lust devil and it left immediately. He said he felt the devil leave. He felt a relief and release of a certain pressure and peace came into his heart. Then in no more than 2 minutes I called the A.I.D.S. devil out and it left immediately. That was in 1990. DB has enjoyed a monogamous heterosexual life ever since and goes to church with his wife and children. The family has supported this ministry around the world. They live in a large southern city.

Case # 9

Pat, a Baptist who contacted the HIV virus from a blood transfusion during surgery. After two years, serious symptoms drove her to the doctor who diagnosed HIV virus in advanced stages giving her only a short time to live. She called for prayer for cancer but revealed at our first meeting that she had A.I.D.S. not cancer. I assured her I was not afraid to lay hands on her for I could not get A.I.D.S since I am covered by the Blood of my God. The Lord promised that he is the Lord-Rapha or Healer, who promised to take all sickness away from us. It is his nature to heal. Also, by the stripes laid on the body of Jesus at the Whipping Post, he took and bore all our sicknesses and diseases. After giving her the healing words I laid hands on her and called the A.I.D.S. devil out and it left immediately. Her church would not allow her to testify that she was healed through the ministry of the Gift of Healing. Her doctors were puzzled. They traced others who had transfusions from the same blood donor and they all had the HIV virus. Her doctors refused to give Jesus Christ glory for his healing of A.I.D.S. That was in early 1992 and today she is the picture of health, looks and acts 10 years younger and is on the go every day.

Case # 10

A lady, Betty, with colon cancer, going for surgery in a few days, received ministry and was healed immediately. When she went to the doctors, they could find no colon cancer. That was in 1992. Today, (1995), she is still healed and working every day.

Case # 11

A young boy, age 13, diagnosed with Multiple Sclerosis shortly after birth. Doctors said he'd never walk or talk. Brought to my Healing Seminar in April 1994 in Prince Albert, SK, Canada. He was healed instantly and could breath and walk better instantly. That afternoon, he could run. A letter from his father dated June 1994: "You will recall praying for our 13 year old son, Samuel. It gives me great pleasure to report that he is an altogether different young man. He got 100% on a math test at school - quite an improvement on a child that the doctors told us shortly after he was born that he never walk or talk. He no longer manifests the symptoms of M.S. that we were so fearful of. Praise the Lord!!! The letter is signed, Clarence (the father).

Case # 12

Robert, age 11, with leukemia and brain cancer -Healed instantly. Dismissed by his doctors in Little Rock Children's Hospital as free of cancer. Robert grew an amazing 6 inches within the first 4 months after his miracle healing. He was brought to West Memphis to my meeting for healing. He received ministry along with his mother and stepfather, and the devil of cancer came out immediately. He was declared free of cancer by his doctors a week later. He grew 6 inches in 4 months. I witnessed this unusual phenomenon of growth also when I visited the family a year later.

Case # 13

A youth, age 19, contracted leukemia. I ministered to him in a hospital room and the cancer devil came out immediately. He was dismissed a week later and returned home. His elders, who practice ancestor worship, a form of necromancy, gathered around him and took him through an ancient Cree Indian witchcraft ritual and claimed that the powers of their ritual healed him of the leukemia. He allowed the elders testimony to stand and did not give the Lord Jesus the glory for his healing. After 9 months the cancer came back in a much worse form and he returned to the hospital.

Three elders, came to the hospital and ministered to him in his room and declared him healed. Lee went home and a week later was back in hospital in a worse condition than ever. I was called to his bedside from another state. While in transit, the Spirit of the Lord spoke clearly to me and said, "Do not go to the hospital. Lee will die of this disease. I will not heal him because he turned back to the religion of ancestor worship". Two days later I called the party who summoned me to minister to Lee and told him I did not go to the Hospital. I told him the reason I did not go. The reply was that Lee died the day before, eaten up with cancer.

Case # 14

Rose, a middle age lady had cancer in the last stages with a short time to live. She was brought 300 miles to my meeting. The party arrived late at night. I went at once upon being contacted and informed by her husband of their arrival. Rose received the words of healing and the cancer devil came out instantly. The power of the Spirit of the

Lord fell on her immediately and she spoke in a new and unknown language. She had never heard about this or seen anyone receive the Holy Ghost Baptism. That was March 1993. Her doctors could not explain her complete recovery, but refused to give Jesus the credit and praise.

Case # I5

Yevett Thomas, a girl age 1, at Cross Lake, Manitoba, Canada had leukemia and had lost her hair due to cancer treatment. She was brought to my services and her mother received the healing words. The cancer devil came out of little Yevett instantly. Doctors could find no more trace of cancer. That was in 1990. Today Yevett is a bright healthy little 7 year old girl, normal with no signs of cancer since her miracle of healing by the Lord Jesus.

Case # 16

Little 9 year old Bob - In a coma for 2 weeks from advanced stages of cancer throughout his little body and expected to die at any time. His parents accepted the healing words. I called the cancer devils out of Bob and they left instantly. He showed no signs of his healing at the time of the miracle. However, when I called Bob's father two days later he said, "Rev Bufkin, my little boy is playing in the front yard". I trembled and shook with fear. I thought that if I could bring this kind of miracle by the Gift of Healing words, I owe this gift to the entire world. Words can never express the impact this healing had upon me. Bob's parents couldn't bring themselves to tell the church they attended how their son got such an instant healing. The church had been praying and fasting around the clock for many months for little Bob. So no one ever testified about the Gift of Healing and the words of healing that brought this instant deliverance.

Several months later the parents moved to another state and took Bob to a Hindu MD for his regular check up. They testified to the Hindu about Bob's healing through the Name of Jesus Christ. The Hindu doctor laid his hands on Bob and called a spirit of sickness back into his body, for he would not allow Jesus Christ to get glory and honor from a miracle of healing. A little over two months from that date, Bob died, but not from cancer. I had the honor of preaching his funeral.

At his funeral I delivered this truth. The law of God says that it is appointed unto man once to die. This is an immutable law. The blessing of divine healing by the stripes of Jesus Christ was not given to repeal that law, but only as a temporary stay at best.

Case # 17

Mrs. CS. had breast cancer. I ministered to her and she received instant healing. The pain left and her flesh began to heal for the cancer had eaten her right breast completely off. Her husband was not in favor of my ministry to her. I instructed him to lay his hands on his wife twice daily and say, 'I love you', and then bless her in prayer and confession of his love for her. Thus he refused to do. Upon my next visit he ordered me out of his house, even though his wife and her mother, who lived with them, had called me to come. Mrs. CS. grew weaker even though her flesh continued to heal. She died of a heart attack 2 months later. The cancer did not come back.

Case # 18

Betty (Tupelo MS at that time) had breast cancer and bone cancer. Her husband abused her severely both verbally and physically. He was extremely jealous and constantly accused her of wanting to contact or communicate with other men. He called her vile names. She was not guilty of any of his accusations. After several years of this, Betty developed cancer. Her husband was so jealous he didn't want me to minister to her or lay my hand even on her head. Friends brought Betty to one of my meetings. She received ministry and was immediately healed of both cancers.

Two years later Betty contacted me again and said one of the cancers was apparently coming back and she was very frightened. Her husband had separated from her and was causing her a great deal of distress. As I ministered to Betty in her home, her husband came into the room and cursed at me and threatened me and ordered me out of the house.

However, Betty told me that the house was hers and not his and asked me to stay and continue ministering the word to her. The husband left the room and I continued and Betty was healed. The pain left her body in early 1993 and as of this date, 1995, has not returned.

Case # 19

Jim had brain cancer in the last stages when a friend asked me to see him. Jim was a professor at a small religious university in Jackson MS. His wife, Joan, was strikingly beautiful and a successful real-estate sales lady. Joan was never at home with Jim and their children. Joan's mother would come to the home and care for the children after school each day and weekends. In the course of time, Jim noticed that Joan would stay away from home daily and then when she was at home she never drew upon any emotional support from him. She became as a visitor in the home to Jim. Jim made no demands on her and didn't ask her about her reasons for withdrawal from her dependence upon his love and emotional support.

Joan became more successful in real estate and was constantly thrown into the company of the most successful men in the city. Jim developed cancer but through all his treatment, Joan never altered her schedule to be with him. Even when I came to the home to minister to him, Joan was nowhere around. Upon arriving at the home, Joan's mother let me in the house and filled me in on details. Jim was barely aware that I was in his presence. I gave him the healing words and the cancer devil came out immediately. His healing was dramatic. Jim got up and escorted me to the door as I left. He has been given 2 weeks to live, but in 10 days he gave a lecture at the university where he was employed. Everything went well for about three months. Jim refused to allow me to meet with him for home Bible Studies. He belonged to one of the old line American Denominations which teaches that the days of miracles have passed and they flatly deny the possibility of all miracles. Jim refused to testify to his church or his family or friends about his miracle of healing. Jim told me that one of his doctors was shocked and admitted that his recovery had to be a miracle. Still Jim would not testify that Jesus Christ had healed him and give the Lord the glory for his recovery. Three months later, Jim developed symptoms of the cancer once again. He died 3 days after his initial examination.

The cancer burst his skull and grew out his nose and ears. NOTE: Healing the wound that caused the cancer is a very urgent necessity. I will help you do this. Call immediately or write.

Case # 20

Little 12 month old baby boy, Adam, had liver cancer which had eaten to the outside of his body. The doctors had destroyed his kidneys with radiation and chemotherapy treatments. A relative who was a doctor (D.C.) picked me up and took me to the home. Three of the grandparents were very opposed to my coming. They did not believe in miracles. One grandmother was present and held Adam as I ministered to him. First I gave the young parents the words of life and healing. They repented and prayed the sinner's prayer and gave their hearts to the Lord. Then I called the cancer devil out of Adam and it left immediately. Unknown to me, the kidneys were healed perfectly at that time also.

The doctors were amazed and the first thing they said was that Adam would not have to have a kidney transplant - that his kidneys were working normally. Then they noticed the cancer and said it was dead except for a tiny spot at the center of the tumor. They wanted to continue chemotherapy and they took full credit for the healing and recovery. However, the cancer was dead instantly when the cancer devils left Adam's body. The doctors were so in unbelief and shock about a liver cancer dying and drying up, they cut into Adam's body to look with their own eyes. The cancer was dead. Doctors will not give the Lord Jesus Christ the glory for healing. They said liver cancers never just go away. BUT faith over ruled facts.

They insisted that their chemotherapy had sent Adam's cancer into remission and to keep it from coming back they must give him several more months of chemotherapy I advised strongly against it but the grandparents and doctors prevailed. The young parents had never seen a miracle and had never been taught how to trust the Lord.

However, Adam received his miracle healing from deadly liver cancer and destroyed kidneys in 1994. Today, (1995), Adam is still pronounced free of cancer and his little kidneys, destroyed completely by the doctor's radiation and chemotherapy, are working normally. It is sad, that Medical Science sees this Gift as being in competition with their work. And miracles are free of charge.

Case # 21

Betty had cancer in her throat in 1994. She came to a church in Tupelo MS where I was ministering and after receiving the words of life she was healed completely. In 2000, she is still healed and rejoicing for her miracle. In October 2009, Betty was still free of cancer and rejoicing in the Lord.

Case # 22

Annie B. had cancer on her kidney in 1994. She called for prayer and received the message about the Cross and Whipping Post. I called the cancer devils out and she was healed instantly. She slept soundly that night. The next day her doctor said the cancer had completely disappeared from her body. In 1995 Annie B. is still praising the Lord for her healing.

Case # 23

A lady in prison in Tupelo MS, had A.I.D.S. The pastor of Good News Church took me there. She received the words about the Cross and Whipping Post, and then prayed the sinner's prayer. I laid my hands on her through the prison bars, called the A.I.D.S. devil out in Jesus Name and it left instantly. Immediately the Holy Ghost fell on her and she spoke in other tongues. She tested HIV negative shortly afterward. Her prison doctors had never had a case of HIV positive suddenly testing HIV negative. That was in 1994. Today, 1995, the lady is out of prison and testifying to her great miracle and going to church regularly. She was released from prison and moved to another state, but still healed.

Case #24

A man from Monroe NC had prostrate cancer problems for 6 years. Finally the cancer spread and doctors gave him up. He came for ministry and heard the truth about the Cross and Whipping Post, prayed the sinner's prayer. When I laid hands on him and called the cancer devils out they came out instantly. He was healed and his doctors, while amazed, pronounced him free of cancer. He reopened his business and went back to work. He testifies to everyone about his healing. A Mr. Hoyle Penegar can verify that miracle healing and many others in that area.

Case #25.

A man named Jeremy was beaten by thugs and left for dead. Doctors pronounced him brain dead. Family asked for help so they put a hose in his throat and forced breathing but said he was brain dead and was only a vegetable and would remain that way for he could not breath on his own. They were going to take the hose out the next day and bury him. An aunt named Mildred took me to his bedside. I had baptized Jeremy 10 months before after he answered an alter call for sinners. I laid hands on his head and said: Devil, I buried this man already in the Name of Jesus Christ. I am not going to let you bury him in the ground. I bound the demons of hate and lust and death and commanded them to come out. WHEN I said the word OUT and raised my hand from his head, he opened his mouth wider that I have ever seen a mouth open and took a long breath. His chest filled out clear to his waist line. Instantly he started breathing on his own. The next day they took him out of the intensive care and a week later he was in rehab and could talk and eat and was alive once again.

Case #26

In 2006, a man named Ron M. in NC contacted a form of paralysis for which there is no medical treatment. The disease was progressing down his back bone from his head. He lost the use of his mouth, tongue, eyelids and arms. He was in the hospital unconscious with a stick in his mouth tied to his tongue so he wouldn't swallow it. Doctors said the paralysis would go to his motor functions at any minute, his heart would stop beating and he would die. I laid hands on him and bound and commanded the paralysis devil to come in Jesus Name. It came out instantly. It smelled like the most rotten meat you ever smelled. After a moment the odor was gone. I then looked at the two other people in the room and gave a prophecy. I said, now tomorrow this man will be sitting up and in a week he will be home.

The next day Ron sat up and wrote the doctor a note. In a week he was home and the next week he was mowing his yard. However, his pastor would not allow him to testify to his miracle. Ron never told anyone about the Lord healing him. I called and wrote him many times but he refused even to meet me or testify to his miracle. Doctors had no explanation for the instant deliverance.

Finally after nearly a year the paralysis started coming back on him. It started in his legs and was going up his body. He refused every request of mine to meet with me for further instruction or to just get acquainted. And his pastor still refused to allow him to testify to the amazing miracle he received.

Case #27

A lady in N.C. named Denise, with inoperable brain cancer came with her husband for ministry. They heard the Word of life and prayed the sinner's prayer. I laid hands on her and called the devils of cancer out and they came out instantly. She was healed. Doctors could find no sign of cancer. However they attended an unbelieving church and the pastor would not allow her to testify to a miracle. When the congregation saw the lady back in church as usual they asked what happened, they all expected her to be dead any time. The pastor said, "Well we all prayed." And he let it go at that, refusing to give the Lord the glory. She never testified to her miracle, though she amazed the doctors and all the neighbors and church members.

Case # 28

A young woman in a University in Arkansas lost her mind when she took an alcoholic drink after taking dope. They kept her in a mental ward locked up for six months. In a meeting at a nearby church they brought her and held her in an area adjoining the church auditorium. During the altar call they brought her to the front row and sat her on the first pew. I stepped down from the platform and whispered in her ear, "Lady, I'm fixing to call that devil out of you." When I spoke to the insane devil and commanded it to leave, she jumped at least 2 feet in the air from a sitting position and screamed like a Banshee Indian. BUT when her feet hit the floor she was speaking in other tongues and weeping. The whole church began to rejoice. Later she married the pastor's son and had two children.

Case #29

A State Representative in Jackson MS brought a man for prayer who was go report to the State Pen the next day to begin a 25 year prison sentence. I prayed for him and then gave him a prophecy. I said, James, you will not serve 5 years of that prison sentence. That was in 1992.

It was 5 years later that the State Rep. came to my home bringing James with a testimony. He said that a weeks before, police had arrested a man in Pascagoula MS for certain crimes. But in the investigation police discovered that this man was guilty of the crimes for which James had been sentenced to prison. The evidence was conclusive and the accused confessed to the crimes thus clearing James completely. When the State Rep heard the news he called the Governor of Mississippi and informed him about the case. Immediately the Governor got on the phone to the State Pen and ordered them to release James and give him financial help. The date…exactly 4 years 10 months after he left my home in 1992.

Case #30

A family in Meridian MS called me for help. Their son had been indicted for felonies in another state and they had posted $40,000 cash bond for him. BUT the trial date was approaching and their son had disappeared. They were frantic that they would lose their $40,000. We went into the Pentecostal church to pray. As soon as we sat down I gave them a prophecy. I said, "Don't worry Mrs. Hughes, the Lord says that in 3 days all charges against your son will be dropped and also, you will get a call from that state saying to come get your $40,000. They will not hold out even a fee." But Mrs. Hughes said, "This is serious…our son could go up for life on this felony charge." I repeated what I just said over again. I said, "Don't worry Mrs. Hughes…" Surely enough in 3 days the charges were dropped and they got a call from the Clerk of Court to come get their $40,000 cash in full.

Case #31

A man I will call Mr. X. a wealthy business man from Le Panto, Arkansas got cancer. His wife called me to come minister to him. Her pastor participated in the interview. I saw that the man was a mocker of the things of the Lord and ridiculed speaking in tongues especially as well as miracles done in Jesus Name. For 30 years he had persecuted his wife and mocked the things of the Lord, especially speaking in tongues. He even mocked speaking in tongues in front of me by babbling. I had never seen anything like it before.

During the night before I was to minister to him the Lord gave me exactly what to say to Mr. X. The next day, I called for the pastor, the wife and children to be there in the bedroom of Mr. X. He was lying in bed when I arrived. Everyone was there. I said, Mr. X. The Lord has been looking at you through a curtain. But the Lord has moved that curtain aside and is laughing at you. You have mocked the things of the Lord for a lifetime. Now the Lord will mock at your calamity. The Lord says you will not rise from that bed of affliction. And I left the room. Mr. X, had never felt he had sinned and never felt the need to repent.

A week later the pastor called saying Mr. X was in a Memphis TN hospital in critical condition. THIS is the only time in my life I have refused to go to a bedside. I said, the Lord said he would not arise from that bed. He died the next day.

Jesus said you could sin against the Father (the Old Testament manifestation of God) and get forgiveness. Jesus said you could sin against the son, Jesus Christ, in the days of his flesh (God manifested in the Son) and get forgiveness. AND it happened exactly like that. The Jewish nation sinned against the Lord Jesus. But Jesus prayed on the cross, Father forgive them, for they know not what they do.

One can never doubt that the greatest sin of the ages, was forgiven in answer to the prayer of the Son of God. They sinned against the Son and got forgiveness.

BUT when you sin against the Holy Ghost (God manifested as the Spirit of Christ) there is no forgiveness in this world or the next. Mr. X sinned for 30 years against the Holy Ghost, which is the Spirit of Christ. He didn't get forgiveness. He is in hell today according to the teaching of the Lord Jesus. That pastor is still there and can confirm every word of this statement.

Case #32

A man named George contacted a very contagious flesh eating virus for which there was no antibiotic. Doctors had him in the top floor of a hospital on the south central part of Little Rock AR. Dr. Frank Slavik, PhD, took me there. No one was allowed in but Dr. Slavik took me in. He leaned against the back wall. I went up to the bed and said. George, don't worry that virus can't get on me. I'm covered by the Blood of my God, the Lord Jesus Christ. George heard the presentation of the Cross and whipping, prayed the sinner's prayer, began weeping when I laid hands on him and called the devil of affliction out of him. It came out instantly. Then I laid hands on George again and said, Receive the Holy Ghost and George began speaking in other tongues. He wept and rejoiced and was healed by the stripes put on Jesus 2,000 years ago. Only a week later they took down the yellow ribbon bands and dismissed George, virus free. His wife was deep into witchcraft.

Case #33

In Cushing, OK a lady had been in a car wreck which killed her husband and left her left leg 4 inches shorter than her right leg. Her bones had been crushed so she was in bad shape. The doctors wanted to amputate her leg but she refused.
I had her try to stamp her foot on the floor saying in Jesus Name. The second time she did it her left leg shot out 4 inches and she screamed. Her healing miracle surprised her. Her left leg was exactly like her right. The miracle stirred many in that area. A year

later she married again to Tippy Burpo.

Case #34

A lady in Prince Albert, Saskatchewan Canada named Helen Black was 28 years old and had grand mal seizures daily for 28 years. Doctors were giving her 5 chemicals to experiment but nothing stopped the seizures. She came to the services in Prince Albert and asked for prayer. She heard about the Blood of Jesus and the stripes. She confessed the sinner's prayer. I laid hands on her head and called the devils by name and bound them and commanded them to come out in Jesus Name. They left immediately. That was in 1994. She never had another seizure. But 4 days later Helen came back to services and received the Holy Ghost baptism just standing in a group of people waiting for prayer. In 2007, she is still healed and doing well.

Case #35

IN early 2006, in N.C., a lawyer's son age 11 had grand mal seizures daily. Nothing doctors could do stopped the horrid epileptic seizures. A man named Hoyle took me to the lawyer's home. I gave the family and the lad the presentation and they all prayed the sinner's prayer. I called the devils out and they left instantly. I calmly told the youth and his family, "The devils are gone - he won't have any more seizures." AND he never had another seizure. I told the family to close every door to demons to reenter by destroying all images especially Walt Disney images from their home. They had baskets full but got rid of them immediately. THE boy has never had another seizure. He runs to hug my neck every time he sees me coming.

Case #36

A secondary school teacher from Grahamstown, South Africa contacted AIDS from her boyfriend. She heard about my ministry in Kenya and got in touch through the web site at http://www.rlbm.org

I mailed her the booklets. She read them and called me. I ministered the word of deliverance by phone and she was healed. During the conversation the Holy Ghost fell on her and she spoke in tongues. That was in 1998. She is still healed today and still teaches in South Africa.

Case #37

A young lady with a drawn up right leg walking with a special crutch came to healing services in Washington, DC area. She came in the altar call hobbling up to the front. But before she got up to me the power of God fell on her and she screamed out. Her crutch went one way and she fell backwards. But before her body hit the floor she was speaking in other tongues. Also, her leg had shot out straight and same length as the other one. That miracle caused a great stir in that area. She walked out holding her crutch above her head pointed up toward heaven. GLORY!

Case #38

A Baptist pastor in N.C. came for help to my home. When he sat down I said…I see you have someone else living inside you. I ministered the word to him and he prayed the sinner's prayer. When I called the devils of deception and witchcraft out of him the Holy Ghost fell on him and he spoke in other tongues. He left a happy and free man. His life was turned completely around. Later his friends told me he was a different man and very happy about his healing miracle.

Case #39

Parents brought their daughter for prayer. Demons would cause her to jerk sometimes violently. She had not slept peacefully for many weeks. After giving the presentation I called the devils out and instantly they left. Her jerking stopped immediately. When they returned to their seat the little girl fell asleep and slept soundly until the next day the parents reported.

Case #40

A man in the hospital in NC was yellow as a pumpkin. It was a form of liver cancer. I told his loved ones that this kind of cancer was much easier than others. They laughed and wondered. I didn't expect them to understand but I wanted to tell them so that after the miracle happened they would believe. Surely enough, the cancer devil came out. Immediately the color of his skin and whites of his eyes changed enough to notice the difference. The next day he was dismissed from the hospital. Doctors had no explanation for liver cancer just doesn't go away. He was healed in Jesus Name.

Case #41

At a church in North Dakota a lady was brought in a wheel chair with MS. She had been that way for years and the doctors said she would never walk again. She along with many others had to wait in the foyer of the church. I got to her and called the MS devils by name, commanded them to come out and they left instantly.

About 6 weeks later as I left Canada I stopped by ND to see the pastor. While in a restaurant a blond lady with a brief case came by and spoke to the pastor. I didn't recognize her. When she left the pastor said, "Did you know that woman?" I said, "Not that I know of." THAT is the lady in the wheel chair, whom doctors said would never walk again. She is selling insurance all over Dickinson. GLORY!

Case #42

A man with skin cancers covering both his arms from his elbows to his wrists came to the healing service for ministry. After giving the Word of life about the Cross and whipping post, he said the sinner's prayer. I called the cancer devils out and they left instantly. There was no immediate sign of his healing. BUT the very next night he came showing his arms. Both arms were clear of cancer sores. There were slight circular marks barely visible as testimony to this miracle.

Case #43

A lady who had both kidneys replaced grew immediately worse. Her body rejected both kidneys. She was passing blood and in pain no medication could abate. Doctors said there was no hope and she would die in about a week or less. Her husband drove her over 100 miles to get to my healing services.

As she came forward and repeated the sinner's prayer, I laid hands on her and commanded the devil of kidney affliction to come out. Instantly the Holy Ghost fell on her and she started speaking in other tongues. Her face flushed red, her pain and bleeding stopped instantly.

She praised the Lord in another language for a long time. Then went to her seat and took her two sons and husband by the hands and brought them for prayer. They prayed the sinner's prayer and rejoiced over the great miracle. Later doctors were baffled at the miracle and admitted it was a miracle. BUT the greatest mystery was, the stitches had disappeared. Glory! The Lord gave her two new kidneys.

Case #44

A man had a friend in the mental ward at Royal Canadian Hospital in down town Montreal. He asked me to go cast the devil out of him. As we entered the large institution we had to wait and be searched and questioned. They took us through large metal doors and again we waited. Then later they took us through another large metal door to a small room with a long table and some chairs. There was a small window in the door where we were watched constantly.

Then they brought the patient in, a Mr. Smith. He sat down and I talked to him for a short time and then laid hands on him and called the insane devils by name and commanded them to come out. Some of them came out. Two more times I called demons out and they finally all came out. I gave him literature as quickly as I could for we were only allowed 20 minutes with him. Then a week later we heard they had taken Mr. Smith out from behind the second set of steel doors. The next week they brought him out into the main open hospital and dismissed him. He is normal in every way today. That was in 2003.

Case # 45

At a tent meeting in Yorkton, Saskatchewan, Canada, they brought a woman who had lost her mind years before. Her head was always tilted to the side and she would not look anyone in the eye. At the altar call she was brought and I called the insane devils out and they left instantly. She shook like she had been hit by a truck and fell backwards. The devils tore her on their way out. She was delivered and received the Holy Ghost and spoke in a heavenly language. Her healing caused a great stir in that city. Multitudes were brought to saving faith in Jesus Christ and also healed as a result of this testimony.

Case # 46

In Nanyuki, Kenya, five women dragged a screaming insane woman to my motel room late one afternoon. I commanded the devils to shut up and come out of her in Jesus Name. I would not allow them to talk. They came out instantly. The woman made a bodily exercise like a snake uncurling. But when she raised her head she spoke perfectly Swahili and was totally sane and thanked the Lord for her deliverance. The entire area was so stirred that many people came to worship and serve the Lord Jesus.

IN 18 years since that fasting I did in that cabin in 1989, many thousands have been saved and healed of every known disease and demon oppression. If you need help get in touch with me immediately. See the contact information at the end of this book. Praying for you in Jesus Name. This update was in December 2007.

UPDATE in 2009   In 20 years of traveling to three continents and uncounted hospitals and sick rooms, there have been more than 550,000 people healed of AIDS and Cancer and every known disease. A very conservative estimate.

The most beautiful results however, is the great number of people, who, either experiencing the miracle working power of Jesus Christ themselves or being witness to the miracles of healing, have, as a direct results of the miracles been brought to faith in the Lord Jesus Christ and are baptized in water by total immersion in the Name of Jesus Christ, and baptized by Jesus with the Holy Ghost as evidenced by their speaking in languages they never learned as the Spirit of Jesus gave them the utterance.

When I saw Jesus face to face, I saw All in All. His image is burned on my mind until I see him again in the rapture or resurrection. Glory!

I give Jesus all the praise. This ministry is not about ME, it is all about the Lord Jesus Christ who is Immanuel, GOD WITH US. It is not about healing; it is really about salvation for the soul.

SPECIAL NOTE:

This Gift of Healing, from the Lord Jesus Christ, emptied the A.I.D.S. wards and the cancers ward at Meru Regional Hospital, Meru, Kenya; East Africa in February 1994. Call Meru General Hospital to verify these many miracles. Ask for Dr. Joseph Mathee. He opened the door to that hospital. There were 10 people in the A.I.D.S. ward and 22 people in the cancer ward. All of the A.I.D.S victims were dismissed as free of A.I.D.S. by March of 1994. Of the 22 cancer patients, one died two days after my visit. But all 21 of the other cancer victims were dismissed from the hospital as free of cancer within a few weeks after my visit. The entire staff, including the nurses and doctors, have notified me that they want me to come back a soon as possible. Read the Nurses own statement on my web site: www.rlbm.org

The doctors at Meru Hospital reported that, "Three weeks after Rev. Bufkin ministered at our hospital, our hospital is 80 percent emptied and we are dismissing patients daily in groups." In 2 days I went to 1,988 hospital beds.

<u>When I bind the devil of cancer or AIDS or witchcraft curses or epilepsy, it is coming out, I don't care what you believe, or if you are unconscious. BUT when you are healed, you must praise the Lord Jesus for healing you and ONLY then will you stay healed and by taking heed to the instructions in this booklet.</u>

If any doubt or pain returns, go to the page with the circle around the Name of the Lord Jesus Christ and lay your hand over the Name of Jesus and repeat the faith confession written below the circle. Stand on the Word of God and you will keep your healing. Notice: Satan and everyone in your world will try to take your healing away by making you doubt. Just confess the Word in return every time they try to make you doubt and you will WIN the spiritual warfare against sickness and disease and all of Satan's temptations.

Dear Pastor Robert L. Bufkin,
I'm a Kenya Government Enrolled Community Nurse working at the Kenyas Infectious Diseases Hospital, Nairobi Kenya.
This is the hospital where all people with infectious diseases are brought in Kenya.
My husband is a senior officer with the Kenya Airforce. I'm pleased to hereby give you a report about what happened after you visited our hospital on 10.2.96 and prayed for 31 patients who had A.I.D.S and T.B. Let me first tell you that you made History to come to our hospital and lay your hands on AIDS patients. No preacher has ever come to lay hands on people who are HIV positive. After your visit, immediately we started seeing changes on most of the patients. We can confess that we stated seeing the changes with the first people you prayed for.
Do you remember the ward where you prayed for 4 patients who could not come out of the ward? Do you remember that when you were there no nurse came inside that room? We could not come because of fear but this is where things started, we could not believe our eyes because within just few hours, three out of the four patients could now sit one died the next day but the three were discharged exactly one week after your visit.
Praise the Lord!
In two weeks, we had discharged almost all of the 30 patients. Out of these were 6 prisoners who were discharged almost immediately.
Let me tell you that we who are in the medical profession don't give any credit to God for healing but since I am the one who was treating these patients before you came and I followed them after you prayed for them, I have seen it better to give the Lord Jesus Christ the Glory and Honor for the healings because He came when we had failed.
Now the six wards in block one which the power of God emptied are now full again with new patients. Please we are requesting you to plan to come as quickly as possible so that these people can also be healed and also you go to more wards.
As we continue with our work, we who know the Lord Jesus, we try to tell the patients about the Lord Jesus Christ.

Wishing you God's blessings as you continue to preach Jesus and bring deliverance to the whole world.

God bless you and remember to pray for us.

Yours in Christ Jesus,

Mrs Esther Kinyanjni.

This next page is of great importance. Say this My Daily Confession Sheet out loud twice a day for 21 days. It will transform your life. Just Try It**. Before you get to the last lines you will sense a peace and assurance coming over you**.

MY DAILY CONFESSIONS

REMEMBER: THE WORDS THAT YOU SPEAK - ARE THE
LANDMARKS OF YOUR LIFE

LORD JESUS, WITH ALL MY HEART, I FORGIVE ALL MY
ENEMIES, I FORGIVE EVERYONE WHO HAS EVER HURT ME,
I TRULY LET THEM GO.
I AM TRULY SORRY FOR ALL MY SINS, I TURN FROM ALL SIN
AND ASK YOU TO FORGIVE ME NOW. I CLAIM THE BLOOD
OF JESUS CHRIST OVER MY SOUL. THERE IS NOTHING IN
MY PAST LIFE THE BLOOD DOESN'T COVER. HEAVEN HAS
NO MORE RECORD THAT I EVER SINNED.
I KNOW THAT JESUS WILL NEVER CHANGE HIS OPINION
ABOUT ME. I WORSHIP YOU JESUS WITH ALL MY HEART.
YOU ARE MY LORD AND MY GOD, MY SAVIOR AND MY
HEALER.

I LOVE YOU JESUS - WITH ALL MY HEART
SAYING IT SOWS IT
I LOVE YOU JESUS - WITH ALL MY MIND
SAYING IT GROWS IT
I LOVE YOU JESUS - WITH ALL MY SOUL AND BODY
SAYING IT KNOWS IT

SATAN: YOU CAN'T GET ABOVE ME - FOR HE COVERS ME
WITH HIS WINGS.
SATAN: YOU CAN'T GET UNDER ME - FOR I'M STANDING
ON HIS EVERLASTING ARMS.
SA TAN: YOU CAN'T GET AROUND ME - HIS ANGELS ARE
CAMPING ALL AROUND ME
AND SATAN: YOU CAN'T CROSS THE ANGELS CAMP
GROUND, GLORY TO GOD!
SATAN: I'M KIN FOLKS TO JESUS CHRIST, RELATED BY HIS
BLOOD, AND
SATAN: YOU CAN'T CROSS THE BLOOD LINE!
PRAISE THE LORD!

MY BODY IS THE TEMPLE OF THE HOLY GHOST. THERE IS NO ROOM FOR SICKNESS OR PAIN OR <u>DEMON SPIRITS OF INFIRMITY. JESUS CHRIST ROSE FROM THE DEAD.</u>
IT IS WRITTEN: JESUS TOOK MY SICKNESS. I DON'T WANT IT BACK; I DON'T HAVE TO HAVE IT. YOU SPIRIT OF SICKNESS AND FEAR, I BIND YOU IN JESUS NAME AND COMMAND YOU TO COME OUT OF MY BODY AND ENTER NO MORE. I PLEAD THE BLOOD OF JESUS CHRIST OVER MY SOUL AND BODY. GO SPIRITS OF OPPRESSION. GET OUT AND STAY OUT IN JESUS NAME. BY <u>HIS STRIPES I'M HEALED   I LOVE YOU JESUS WITH ALL MY HEART!</u>

I AM GROWING MORE INTO THE IMAGE OF JESUS CHRIST BY OBEDIENCE TO HIS WORD!
I CAN DO ALL THINGS THROUGH CHRIST WHO STRENGTHENS ME, FOR IT IS WRITTEN: GREATER IS HE THAT IS IN ME, THAN HE THAT IS IN THE WORLD. LORD JESUS, I WILL READ YOUR WORD AND PRAY. I WILL OBEY YOUR WORD. I WILL FOLLOW YOU JESUS ALL MY LIFE. BAPTIZE ME WITH THE HOLY GHOST. I WILL RAISE MY HANDS AND PRAISE YOU LORD JESUS. I WILL TESTIFY TO MY MIRACLE. I WILL SPEAK YOUR HOLY NAME OVER ALL MY PAIN AND TROUBLES!

I OVERCOME EVIL WITH GOOD. I OVERCOME SATAN AND TEMPTATION BY THE BLOOD OF THE LAMB AND THE WORD OF MY TESTIMONY. LIKE ENOCH, I CONFESS THAT, "<u>I PLEASE GOD</u>".

TAPE THIS PAGE TO YOUR MIRROR <u>CONFESS IT OUT LOUD TWICE DAILY FOR 21 DAYS</u>. YOU WILL FEEL A SURGE OF PEACE AND CALM COME IMMEDIATELY INTO YOUR HEART. IT WILL TURN SADNESS INTO JOY, DEPRESSION INTO HAPPINESS, DOUBT INTO FAITH. IT WILL TRANSFORM YOUR LIFE. TRY IT JUST ONCE AND SEE. IT WILL BREAK THE POWER OF DEMON OPPRESSION IF YOU SAY IT FROM YOUR HEART!

Distributed by Rev. Robert L. Bufkin; PO Box 17382; Jonesboro
AR, 72403. 206 203 6273; anelijah@fastmail.fm
Call or write for prayer or for book list. My Books can be ordered
from the web site: http://www.rlbm.org
or the above address or by Email. For home study or Church
ministry get in touch immediately.

IF YOU DESIRE HELP OR COUNSEL – CALL OR WRITE
IMMEDIATELY.

Contact me at: (206) 203-6273

Download our CD:
    "The Gift of Healing Cancer & AIDS"

Free Online – go to www.GiftOfHealingCD.com

Multitudes have been healed all over the world by listening to the
Healing CD and following the simple instructions. You too can be
healed and delivered if you will listen to the simple words on the CD.
But you may call the author at a pre-arranged time and he will
minister the Words of Healing to you personally.

The author travels a great deal to conduct Healing and Deliverance
Seminars all over the US and Canada. If you desire to have his ministry
in your Church or a public building get in touch at the address above.

www.ingramcontent.com/pod-product-compliance
Lightning Source LLC
Chambersburg PA
CBHW020338290526
45785CB00005B/2084